The After 50 Pharmacy

An Easy-To-Understand Guide to Prescription and Nonprescription Medications

Ann and James Kepler with William Swisher, M.D.

CONTEMPORARY
BOOKS, INC.
CHICAGO ▪ NEW YORK

CONTENTS

FOREWORD

We have to consider the age of the person before we can discuss the effects of any drug. To simplify this we can divide older people into the "Young Old," that is, the ages 50 through 65. The "Middle Old" are arbitrarily set at 65 to late 70s, and the "Old Old" are those over 75.

The "Young Old" person handles drugs much like any adult. His or her body makeup is about the same, and usually the organ systems still have considerable reserve capacity to handle disease, drugs, and the stressful crises of living.

After 65 the changes we associate with aging become manifest, although they have been going on for a few decades. The relationship of muscle to fat changes with loss of muscle and perhaps accumulation of fat. The serum protein tends to be less. Thus, drugs that are bound to protein do not have the same amount of protein to adhere to as in the younger person, so the free drug may easily reach toxic levels. The fat soluble drugs accumulate in the fat and build up and remain in the body after we would like to be rid of them.

Medicine taken by mouth may not be absorbed as well in the older person for several reasons. There may be a change in the acidity of the stomach, the digestive juices may not be as powerful, or the blood supply to the digestive tract may be impaired.

Drugs are usually excreted by the kidneys or broken down into harmless by-products by the liver. In the "Middle Old" people these organs may have little more than one-third the capacity of younger adults, so the older person takes longer to rid the body of drugs. Of course, if either the liver or kidneys are diseased, this process takes much longer.

By the time a person is in his or her late 70s or older, there is little or no reserve left. He or she may do quite well when life is normal, but find it increasingly difficult to handle disease, the medicine used to treat the disease, or any other form of stress.

Dosages of most medicines must be lower as the person ages, and that is one reason doctors need to see the older patient from time to time to determine if he or she is still tolerating a long-continued medicine. The doctor who is trained or experienced in the care of the older person will usually start out prescribing about one-fourth the usual adult dose. Often about one-half the full dose will produce the same effect in the very old that a full dose will in a younger person.

The older person usually needs to take more than one medicine because he or she has more than one condition that needs treatment. If two drugs are detoxified by the same enzyme in the liver, there will not be enough enzyme to detoxify both drugs so a toxic level may easily build up.

Drugs today are potent, and dosage is important. Do not take more than the doctor prescribed because there is often a narrow margin between the desired effect and the toxic effect. Do not omit a dose or take less than the doctor prescribed because this may prevent the medicine from doing what it is supposed to do. Of course, if a reaction is thought to occur that might be harmful, it is wise to discuss immediately the matter with your doctor. It is important to talk with your doctor if you have any changes that you can't explain. You should know the main side effects or the effects of toxic levels of any drug and watch for them.

William Swisher, M.D.

AN IMPORTANT NOTE TO READERS

Every effort has been made to present the information in *The After-50 Pharmacy* in the most accurate manner. However, this book is not intended to take the place of your doctor or pharmacist. Different people—and this applies especially to older persons—may react differently to the same medication, course of treatment, or procedure. Always consult your doctor before undertaking any course of treatment or drug therapy.

Neither the authors, the consultant, nor the publisher takes responsibility for any potential consequences following any action, procedure, or administration of medication by anyone reading and following the suggestions in this book. Drug research and developments change constantly in the pharmaceutical industry, and you are urged to consult your physician, pharmacist, or other health-care professional for the latest advice on specific subjects or drugs.

The inclusion of a drug or product, either prescription or nonprescription and listed by either brand name or generic name, does not constitute an endorsement of that drug or product. Conversely, the exclusion of a drug or product is not a statement that that drug or product is ineffective or unsafe. Space and the scope of this book necessarily limit the number of products included. Since there are hundreds of drugs on the market, including many that have similar uses, this book has been limited to those drugs most commonly prescribed. If the drug your doctor prescribed is not in this book, you may find a general discussion of that kind of drug in Chapter 3.

PART I: THE AFTER-50 PHARMACY

1

HOW TO USE THIS BOOK

Perhaps you have sometimes wondered about questions such as these:

- When is it safe for me to take an over-the-counter drug?
- How do I decide on the dosage?
- What questions should I ask the doctor about my prescription?
- How can I recognize side effects that I may develop from prescription or nonprescription medicines?
- How do I know if I really need to take any medicine? Don't some ailments just go away by themselves?
- What kinds of medical supplies should I keep on hand?
- How can I find out if drugstore patent remedies are any good?
- Is there specific information I should be aware of when I buy and use prescription medicines?

At some time or another, everyone is faced with some kind of illness. If the complaint is minor, you may simply deal with it at home. When the problem is more serious, however, you generally turn to a physician or another health-care professional for help. In either case, you often must take medications, and your ability to make sensible decisions about drugs—either nonprescription or prescription—may mean the difference between an uneventful recovery and a prolonged illness.

The After-50 Pharmacy is a personal guide to medications. It consists of two sections: general information about taking medications, followed by a series of profiles of specific and commonly used prescription and over-the-counter (OTC) medicines. The latter section contains notes on dosage forms and strengths, facts about signs of possible overdose, and other information.

Within the following pages you'll find answers to questions ranging from "When should I take—or not take—aspirin?" to "How will I recognize a potentially harmful reaction to a prescription?" The goal is to provide you with enough facts to become a responsible, knowledgeable, and effective caretaker of your own health.

Maybe you often use over-the-counter remedies to treat your minor illnesses. Generally, about the only guidance you get on a regular basis regarding these products is advertising claims. Just how accurate are they? The best way to find out is to ask questions of your doctor and your pharmacist. Some remedies are very helpful, and some are simply not worth the expense. Check the guidelines provided in Chapters 2 and 4 for selecting medicine-cabinet supplies and OTC preparations, and then, before making a purchase, discuss the product with your druggist. (Don't rely on the opinions and personal experiences of the drugstore clerk, by the way. Talk to a registered pharmacist; he or she has been trained specifically to know the composition and actions of drugs. Even OTC preparations can cause serious problems if used incorrectly.)

Many widely advertised OTC medications (also called *patent remedies*) may provide slight relief of minor symptoms, but their overall effectiveness is minimal. A few can even do more harm than good. Perhaps some of the medicines that your own parents used to treat you when you weren't well are still on the market and selling well. That fact alone, however, does not mean that those products are either effective or entirely safe.

You should always check with either your doctor or your pharmacist before taking any kind of OTC remedy. There is no point in wasting your money, and you certainly don't want to risk making your condition worse than it already is. If a product with which you are familiar is not listed in Part II of this book, ask a health-care professional's advice before buying it. It could be that the item does not measure up to its advertised claims, or perhaps there is another, more beneficial product that would do the job better, faster, or cheaper. Of course, with the hundreds of products on the market, some item's omission from the profile list does not mean that it is ineffective or harmful.

Because not all medications are used to treat or cure illness—some are designed to prevent illness—Chapter 8 tells you how to stay healthy by taking advantage of immunizations and food supplements. You'll also find useful information about a common disease of older women called *osteoporosis* in this chapter.

Aspirin and aspirin substitutes are the most commonly used OTC medications, and you will find helpful information on those drugs in Chapter 2. Such topics as aspirin freshness and the advisability of using aspirin while taking other medicines are discussed.

Prescription drugs, by their very nature, are used under a doctor's orders. Nevertheless, the more you understand about prescription drugs, the more likely it is that you will be able to comply knowledgeably with your doctor's instructions. Research has shown that many persons, upon leaving their doctor's office, do not fully understand what the doctor has told them about using a prescribed drug. When you turn to Chapter 5, you will learn how to read a prescription and how to have it filled. Included is a list of questions to ask your doctor before taking any prescription drug. And keep in mind that there is nothing wrong with asking your physician whether or not you really need a prescribed medication.

Whether you are treating your ailment with over-the-counter or prescription medications, you will need to know how to select and take various forms of drugs. How can you accurately measure liquid medicine so that you don't take too much? How can you avoid potentially harmful food or drug interactions when you are taking a variety of different medicines? Chapter 7 will help you avoid hazardous situations.

Being aware of and coping with possible drug side effects is also your responsibility. But which side effects are minor and expected, and which are serious adverse reactions? When can you handle a minor side effect, and when should you call your doctor? Chapter 6 will help you become alert to both major and minor drug reactions as you treat your illness. Knowing what to watch for is an important part of assessing the effectiveness of the treatment process.

Older persons often take a wide variety of drugs, and Chapter 3 discusses in detail precisely how several families of drugs work. Many medicines that formerly were relied on as pharmaceutical staples have now been replaced by more effective and safer drugs. Knowledge of the ways in which medications function as they help control or prevent disease is essential if you are effectively to help your doctor manage your illnesses.

Chapter 9 offers some helpful tips for those who may be caregivers of their spouses, parents, or other relatives. It is unfortunate but true that most persons who find themselves in such situations often have little or no training or experience to help them cope with their new responsibility.

The profiles of drugs in Part II—both prescription (Chapter 10) and over-the-counter (Chapter 11)—that are commonly used for treating illnesses in older persons are listed alphabetically within each chapter for easy reference. Check them for warnings regarding specific medications as well as for storage and administration tips, side effect and overdose symptoms, and helpful precautions and suggestions. The profiles of OTC products also include recommended dosages.

Remember that all modern drugs are powerful and affect the way your body functions. The proper dose is important because too much of a drug can be toxic and too little can be ineffective. Before you take them into your body, you should learn all you can about them. The purpose of this book is to help you do just that. Don't hesitate to ask questions of your physician, pharmacist, or any other health-care professional. It's important that you learn all you can about your medicine so that you can use it most effectively to heal, not to harm.

2

YOUR HOME
MEDICAL CENTER

You can establish a medical center in your home that is efficient, reliable, and safe. The things to keep in mind are simplicity and orderliness. You might want to set aside a roomy shelf or two in a linen closet or cupboard outside the bathroom. This area, combined with your bathroom medicine cabinet, should allow ample space for your basic medical needs.

Use your bathroom cabinet only for a few first-aid supplies and basic health and medical equipment. Unless you or a member of your family has a specific need for certain kinds of medical appliances or medicines, it is unlikely that you will need anything beyond a few staple items. A cluttered cabinet filled with several different brands of the same item or old, outdated, or little used products makes it difficult for you to find what you need in a hurry. And, of course, there is the very real chance that you may need to do just that. You

might not have the time to search among a variety of boxes and bottles to find what you need in an emergency.

YOUR BATHROOM
MEDICINE CABINET

A bathroom cabinet should properly be used to store only toiletries, first-aid supplies, and a few nonprescription products that you may need on a day-to-day basis. Do not keep prescription medications there. The heat and steam of the bathroom can have a harmful effect on them. Also, if there are small children living in or visiting your home, it is best not to keep medications or solutions of any kind, including those you purchase without a prescription, in the medicine cabinet. Children can be very quick; they can climb up on a washbasin and reach into a cabinet in the time it takes you to answer the telephone or check something on

Poison Control Centers

Check your telephone directory now for the number of the poison control center nearest you; it should be listed under "Poison." If there is no listing, call your nearest hospital emergency room and ask for the number. Post the number permanently on each of your telephones or on the wall near each telephone. Taking this action now may save your life or the life of someone else who accidentally swallows too much or the wrong kind of medicine or spills a caustic substance on his or her skin.

The poison control center will likely have a toll-free 800 number. That may or may not mean that the center is located in another city. Don't be concerned if the center is not local; it is still your best source of information concerning poisons. Occasional efforts have been made to establish a single national source for all information about poisons, but as yet the United States has no central clearinghouse for such data. Therefore, regional centers have been designated to supply vital information to hospitals, health-care professionals, fire and police departments, and the general public.

If you telephone the center in an emergency and say, "I think I just took too much medicine," the first question you will be asked will be "What was it and how much did you swallow?" Be prepared to answer by taking the container with you to the telephone. Tell the center the name of the drug if you know it. If you don't know the name, state your name, the name and telephone number of the drugstore where the prescription was filled, the prescription number, and your doctor's name. If the medicine was not a prescription, read the name of the medicine from the label and tell the center what the list of ingredients says is in it. Tell the center if you are taking any other kinds of medicine, even though you may not have taken too much of another kind.

Describe any symptoms you are experiencing and be ready to write down whatever instructions the center gives you. You may be told how to treat the problem yourself or that you are in no danger and do not need to take any action. Or the center may instruct you to call an emergency squad or your doctor. Be certain you clearly understand each instruction and then do exactly what you are told to do.

Aspirin Freshness

Sometimes, after repeated exposure to the air, aspirin tablets may decompose chemically, although they appear normal. Each time you open a bottle of aspirin, sniff the contents. An odor resembling vinegar indicates that the chemical composition of the aspirin has broken down and that the aspirin is not safe to use. When this happens, discard the contents by flushing the unused tablets down the toilet, and buy a new bottle. Because of aspirin's tendency to decompose rather quickly, it is often better for you to purchase small-quantity bottles rather than "economy" sizes. When it becomes necessary to throw away part of what you have bought, the per-tablet savings you thought you made by buying the larger size are lost.

the stove. Many medications, with their brightly colored packages and containers, appear attractive to children, and their curiosity could lead to a dangerous situation. Medications should be kept in a locked cabinet if there are children in your home.

Basic supplies for your medicine cabinet might include the following items.

Pain Relievers

Aspirin is the most commonly used analgesic, or pain reliever, and is sold under various trade names, such as Bayer and St. Joseph's, as well as generically, when it is sometimes called *acetylsalicylic acid*, or *ASA* for short. Aspirin was perhaps the first "wonder drug" and has been in common usage for more than half a century. Its strength is indicated in terms of grains or milligrams (mg). Adult-strength aspirin is 5 grains, or 325 mg, per tablet. A normal dosage is two tablets for minor headache or pain, to be repeated after four hours if the discomfort persists. As with many other medications, however, the amount of aspirin needed by different individuals varies according to their body size. That is to say that, while one or two tablets may quickly relieve the discomfort of someone weighing 100 pounds, the dosage would probably need to be increased for another person weighing 275 pounds.

Aspirin is an excellent remedy for symptomatic relief of pain and discomfort and has so few side effects that it may be used widely and safely by most people. This is not to say, however, that some persons do not exhibit adverse reactions to the drug. There are some instances, within a relatively small percentage of the population, when severe problems can develop from the use of aspirin. It is likely that an adult would be aware of his or her sensitivity to the drug simply because of its wide and continued popular usage, but it is also possible for a reaction to even such a common medication to appear suddenly despite previous uneventful usage. As the body ages, changes sometimes occur that cause new reactions to certain foods and medicines that formerly could be enjoyed and used with impunity. Many such new sensitivities can also be attributed to interactions between previously commonly used foods or drugs and a new or different kind of prescription medication never taken before. For this reason it is essential that you tell your physician exactly what procedure you follow to treat minor headaches and occasional aches and pains. If your treatment involves the use of aspirin, he or she may caution you about its continued usage. Ask your doctor about the effects of prolonged use of aspirin.

For some of those persons for whom aspirin is not recommended, an aspirin substitute called *acetaminophen* is often effective. Acetaminophen is sold generically as well as under such trade names as Tylenol and Panadol. It is available in the same strength as aspirin, that is, 5 grains, or 325 mg, per tablet, and it is to be taken in the same dosages and on the same schedule as aspirin, two tablets at four-hour intervals.

Recently a new pain reliever called *ibuprofen* has appeared on the over-the-counter market. Formerly sold only with a doctor's order as the prescription drug Motrin, ibuprofen is now available in a weaker strength as nonprescription remedies such as Advil and Nuprin. Unlike aspirin or acetaminophen, ibuprofen is sold in 200-mg tablets and should generally be taken one tablet at a time at four- to six-hour intervals for pain. Ibuprofen should not be taken by persons who have ever had an allergic reaction or sensitivity to aspirin.

Aspirin, acetaminophen, and ibuprofen are all effective for the treatment of pain and fever, but aspirin and ibuprofen have an additional effect against inflammation—the redness, heat, and soreness that appear around cuts, bruises, and damaged tissues. Acetaminophen may help ease some of the pain of inflammation but will do little to relieve the redness or swelling. None of these

Ibuprofen Warnings

Do not take ibuprofen (Nuprin, Advil) if you are also taking aspirin or if you have any sensitivity to aspirin.

Ask your doctor whether you should take ibuprofen for minor pain. While you are talking to the doctor, ask him or her whether a prescription for this drug would be cheaper. The prescription versions of ibuprofen, Motrin and Rufen, have been reduced in price by their manufacturers to compete with the OTC versions. However, the prescription formulations still have a higher dosage of medication and, therefore, may be unsuitable for some persons.

products will kill any germs that may be helping to cause some of the inflammation.

Keep in mind that dosages for pain relievers, as for many other kinds of drugs, are based on body size. But adults come in all shapes and sizes. It may be that a single aspirin tablet will suffice for the relief of a severe headache suffered by a small person, while two or even three tablets are needed by a very large person. It is a good idea to discuss medication dosages, including those of over-the-counter drugs, with your physician. Your pharmacist also is a good resource for information about nonprescription remedies.

Antacid

Avoid the fizzy types of antacid. They are very high in so-dium and actually add more acid to an already upset stomach. Turn instead to milky-appearing liquids such as Mylanta, Gelusil, Maalox, or a wide variety of others, including generic "house brands" sold by large pharmacy chains. The tablet forms of these medicines are effective as well and are convenient to carry along with you when you're away from home. One tablet form, Tums, has an extra bonus: it contains calcium and thus provides extra calcium for bone strength. It has been estimated that 40 percent of people over 70 years of age do not get adequate calcium in their diet, and, therefore, the use of an antacid such as Tums boosts calcium intake.

Antacids are not all compounded in the same way. They may have bases of aluminum, zinc, magnesium, or a combina-

What You Should Know About Aspirin

With millions of tablets being consumed every day, aspirin is by far the most familiar and commonly used over-the-counter remedy. Since it is so easily available and such a widely used drug, it is sometimes taken for granted. Aspirin, however, should not be dismissed lightly as just another household product. It has very real medical properties and should be treated with the same degree of caution as other drugs.

- If you bleed easily or have an ulcer, check with your doctor before taking aspirin or any product containing aspirin.
- If you are sensitive to aspirin, use an aspirin substitute containing acetaminophen, such as Tylenol or Panadol. Do not, however, use a product, such as Advil or Nuprin, that contains ibuprofen.
- Read the labels of all nonprescription medicines you are currently using to see whether aspirin is one of the ingredients. Remember that aspirin as one ingredient of a compound may be identified by its chemical name, acetyl-salicylic acid, or ASA for short. Taking a couple of aspirin tablets along with another medicine, a cold remedy, for example, could result in an aspirin overdose. Ask your pharmacist's advice if you are unsure about the aspirin content of various products.
- Be certain to inform your doctor if you are taking aspirin, even occasionally, as a painkiller. It could have an effect on the type of medicine he or she prescribes for you.
- Drink at least one full glass (eight ounces) of water each time you take aspirin and at least six to eight during the day. Increase that amount if you have a fever or if you have a disease for which your doctor has prescribed daily aspirin therapy.
- Do not exceed the manufacturer's recommended dosage without your physician's advice.
- If you have asthma, ask your doctor whether you should take aspirin.
- If aspirin causes you to have an upset stomach, ask your physician or pharmacist to recommend an aspirin product that has a coating that will prevent the tablets from dissolving until after they leave your stomach.

- If you begin to experience dizziness, ringing or buzzing in your ears, an unusual thirst, or rapid breathing, take no more aspirin and call the poison control center or your doctor immediately. You could be suffering from aspirin overdose. An overdose can occur in some persons who have taken even small amounts of aspirin.

tion of these and other ingredients. You should be aware that some antacids (particularly those containing magnesium) may cause diarrhea, and some (particularly those containing aluminum) may cause constipation. If you are already experiencing one or the other of these conditions, don't make it worse by selecting a product that will only add to your problem. Also, some antacids are available that have sodium-free formulas, especially important for persons who must watch the amount of salt they consume. Discuss your individual need with your pharmacist and ask his or her advice about which antacid may be best for you to stock in your medicine cabinet.

Petroleum Jelly

Sold as Vaseline and under other trade names, including many generic products, petroleum jelly is an inexpensive lubricant that is effective for treating and soothing chapped skin. It is useful as well for lubricating rectal thermometers. (Petroleum jelly should not be used to lubricate any product containing rubber, such as rectal tubes, however, because it will cause them to deteriorate. For those purposes, use a nonpetroleum lubricant called K-Y Jelly, a clear, water-soluble gel sold in tubes in most pharmacies.) Purchase petroleum jelly in tubes if possible, to reduce the risk of contaminating the unused portion of the product, and store it away from heat, which will cause the jelly to melt into a liquid.

Alcohol

Household alcohol is a disinfectant that is useful for cleaning thermometers, glassware, and other hard surfaces to help prevent the spread of germs. It is sold as rubbing alcohol or isopropyl alcohol, generally in a solution strength of about 70 percent. Alcohol used as a rub is soothing to tired or aching muscles. It should not be poured into cuts or open wounds because it can damage delicate tissues and would probably also increase the amount of discomfort already present from the injury. *Rubbing alcohol is poisonous and should never be taken internally.* Remember, too, that it is flammable and should not be used around an open flame, including lighted cigarettes.

Hydrogen Peroxide

Hydrogen peroxide is another inexpensive mild disinfectant that is useful for cleansing cuts and abrasions. Poured directly into a wound, it causes a fizzing or bubbling action that helps lift dirt and debris out of the injured area. It may cause a very slight stinging sensation, but that sensation is only temporary. Peroxide is sold in a solution strength of 3 percent and is always contained in a brown glass or plastic bottle to protect it from light. Continued exposure to light weakens the solution, so peroxide should always be stored in a closed cupboard. The solution tends to deteriorate relatively quickly and should be replaced after three to four months.

Calamine Lotion

A claylike substance called *kaolin* forms the base of calamine lotion. It is mixed with water and, sometimes, zinc oxide to form a soothing lotion that is effective in relieving the itching and stinging of insect bites and irritation from poison oak, ivy, and sumac. Calamine lotion should be applied around and over the affected area with a cotton ball or swab. Use a fresh one each time you need more lotion to prevent contamination; don't touch the bottle with an applicator already used. Do not apply lotion directly to an open, weeping, or crusted sore; in those instances, daub the lotion only around the perimeter of the affected area. As the lotion dries, it forms a white-to-pink powdery coating over the skin. Leave the area open to the air if possible, so that the lotion can dry.

Hydrocortisone Cream

Hydrocortisone is a steroid drug that is beneficial in treating minor skin irritations resulting from poisonous plants, insect bites, and exposure to some soaps and harsh cleaning solutions. It is available in 0.5 percent strength as a cream, ointment, or lotion. Hydrocortisone should be applied in a thin coat over the affected area, gently rubbed in, and allowed to air-dry. After applying, wash your hands immediately so you do not get the medication in your eyes.

Nose Drops

Phenylephrine hydrochloride in a 1 percent solution (Neo-Synephrine is an example) is an effective decongestant product for treating the runny nose symptoms of a common cold. It works by constricting the blood vessels within the nose, thereby reducing congestion. Nose drops should be used for only two to three days because they cause the vessels to tire to the point that they once again begin to dilate, necessitating heavier doses and causing an increase in the amount of secretions. Use beyond three days often leads to a condition worse than that for which treatment was begun in the first place.

FIRST AID SUPPLIES

Everyone experiences minor cuts, scratches, and burns from time to time. Such injuries are seldom troublesome for the person whose overall health is good. But they are painful and annoying and should be treated properly in order to prevent infection and more serious problems. A mild disinfectant such as an iodine solution (select a nonstinging brand such as Betadine) is handy for painting an injured area after thoroughly cleaning it with soap and water and before a protective cover is applied. Don't bother with mercurochrome or merthiolate, by the way; according to the Food and Drug Administration (FDA), they are neither safe nor effective as germicides. A supply of sterile cotton or cotton balls is handy for applying liquids that do not come equipped with applicators.

Keep a supply of adhesive bandage strips on hand to cover small cuts and some sterile, individually wrapped two-inch-by-two-inch gauze pads and adhesive tape for larger injuries. Adhesive tape may be purchased in cloth, plastic, and paper varieties, depending on your preference. The plastic is best if it is likely that the area may become wet, but paper tape is best if you have previously experienced a reaction to adhesives. When applying adhesive tape, be careful not to stretch the tape too tightly or to wrap it all the way around a limb. Incorrectly applied tape can impair circulation and lead to serious circulatory problems. The best method for covering an injury is to lay gauze gently over the area, cut adhesive strips that will extend slightly beyond the gauze, and pat them down on the skin lightly enough to hold the bandage in place but not so tightly that circulation may be hindered. In place of adhesive tape, you might prefer using rolled gauze to hold bandages in place. Again, do not tie the gauze too tightly.

Elastic bandages are useful for supplying support to weakened leg or arm muscles. Care must be taken, however, not to wrap them too tightly because they may impair circulation. Properly applied, an elastic bandage is unrolled as it is wrapped securely around the affected limb. Be sure that you do not stretch the fabric as you apply it so as to avoid binding.

Besides these basic products, you will probably want to have on hand a few additional items, such as the following.

Tweezers

Select tweezers that are blunt-ended and whose ends are well-aligned. They are handy for removing splinters as well as for picking up small items or pulling cotton plugs out of medicine bottles.

Scissors

A small pair of blunt scissors kept in the medicine cabinet at all times is handy for cutting adhesive tape or rolled gauze bandages. Having to look through drawers or cupboards for scissors as you try to secure a bandage can be frustrating.

Medication Spoon

These special spoons are intended for use by children, but they are so handy to use when taking liquid medicines that they should be kept in all medicine cabinets.

Medication spoons are shaped like laboratory test tubes, except a large spoon-shaped extension is added to the open end of the tube. The tube itself is glass or plastic and is marked in medical teaspoon measurements. A medical teaspoon is a precise liquid measure, and, for that reason, a kitchen teaspoon (flatware), which may hold a little more or a little less than a medical teaspoon, should not be used to measure medications. To use a medication spoon, hold the tube at eye level and pour the liquid medicine into it until you reach the prescribed amount. Then place the spoon-shaped end in your mouth and tip the teaspoon up.

Keep in mind that all medicines, even those sold over the counter, should be measured as accurately as possible. You may purchase a medication spoon from most pharmacies.

First Aid Manual

Don't wait until you or someone else in your household suffers an injury to go looking for a book of instructions that will tell you what to do in an emergency. Keep a small booklet in the medicine cabinet that briefly outlines what to do for bruises, cuts, sprains, etc. You might ask your pharmacist to recommend one to you; he or she might even have on hand some complimentary material offered at no cost by a pharmaceutical manufacturer.

Thermometer

Quite often when you telephone your physician to make an appointment for a nonroutine office visit you are asked if a high temperature is one of your symptoms. A temperature elevated above the normal 98.6°F can indicate an infection of some kind. Of course, there is no way you can know for certain whether you have a fever unless you have a thermometer on hand. Therefore, either a common glass oral thermometer or one of the newer electronic thermometers (which, with their large, digital displays, may be easier to read) should be a part of your medicine cabinet equipment.

PRESCRIPTION MEDICATIONS

It is not at all unusual for older persons to be taking as many as half a dozen different prescription and nonprescription medications at the same time. It seems that, as we grow older and our physical health begins to decline, the number of drugs we use increases. Many older persons may be taking mild to moderately strong tranquilizers, antibiotics, aspirin, and perhaps something for heart disease or hypertension. Add to these occasional cold remedies or OTC sleeping pills, and the need for proper and safe storage and administration becomes extremely important.

As stated earlier, it is unwise to store medicines in a bathroom medicine cabinet, where moisture and heat may cause some drugs to deteriorate. Instead, keep them in a cool place away from light. A linen closet near the bathroom is ideal. Of course, if there are young children in the home, all medicines should be kept on a shelf high enough to be out of their reach and, ideally, inside a locked container. Children should never be allowed to watch you take the key from its safe location, unlock a medicine box, and take your medicine. Most children love to imitate adults, and the result could be disastrous. Again, when children are present, even as occasional visitors, medicine bottles should *never* never be left sitting on a kitchen counter or table.

Don't rely on so-called child-proof pill bottles to prevent children from playfully eating brightly colored pills that may appear to them to be the same as candies such as M&Ms. Children often have less trouble opening those bottles than adults do. (Because childproof containers are hard to open by patients with arthritis or little strength in their hands, it may be best to ask the pharmacist to use regular screw-top or snap-lid bottles.)

A small metal or plastic fishing tackle box, toolbox, or artist's supply case makes an excellent medicine container; choose one that has a lock on it. If you find a box that has a compartmentalized tray that raises automatically as the lid is opened, you can use as many spaces as you need for different kinds of medicines and add a few first aid supplies and other useful items to the larger space in the bottom. This arrangement has the advantage of providing a safe storage place for all your drugs and also serves as a traveling medicine chest that is always ready to go when you are. This is especially handy when you go to the doctor. *It is wise to take all of your medications and over-the-counter products with you each time you visit your doctor*, particularly if you are being treated by more than one doctor. This allows the doctor to check the dosage and prevents him or her from giving you another medication that duplicates or interacts with one you are already taking.

Taking this kind of medicine chest from a closet, unlocking it, and picking out your required medicines several times a day may prove to be a nuisance. If that is the case, ask your pharmacist to recommend a medicine container that is divided into seven compartments and designed to hold a week's worth of medicine. Then, once a week, count out all the tablets you will need to take during the upcoming week, and store the remaining supply in your portable medicine chest. Keep your weekly medication container safely out of the reach of visiting or resident children.

If you use the toolbox method of storing your medicines, do not empty the contents of individual pill bottles into the compartments. All medicine supplies should be kept in the original containers that have directions printed on them. Original containers also have tighter-fitting lids that will help keep their contents fresh longer. It is a good idea to label your portable medicine chest or weekly medication container with your name and the name and telephone number of your doctor.

What Is Blood Pressure?

Blood pressure is the force of the blood as it is pumped from the heart and travels throughout the body's blood vessels. In simple terms, it is a measure of the amount of pressure exerted against the vessel walls. The precise strength of that force can be measured only by the use of a medical device called *sphygmomanometer*.

The higher figure of a measured blood pressure is called the *systolic pressure*. (Blood pressure is written as, say, 120/80 and is stated as "one twenty over eighty.") It is the amount of force created within the vessels as the heart contracts and pushes blood out, thus causing it to circulate. *Diastolic pressure*, the lower figure, is measured as the heart relaxes and refills with blood between beats.

Normal blood pressure (the numbers signify the millimeters of mercury raised and recorded on a sphygmomanometer) is approximately 120 (systolic) over 80 (diastolic) in a young, healthy adult. Normal, however, can have different meanings for different people. As we grow older and our vessels acquire inner deposits and lose some elasticity, our pressure may climb slightly. Therefore, a physician must consider many factors when determining what is "normal" blood pressure for an individual. Some of those factors are age, sex (women usually have slightly lower pressure than men), lifestyle (amount of worry and fatigue), and physical build. Another factor is whether a person is overweight. A heavy arm can cause an inaccurate reading; therefore, a special cuff is necessary to measure blood pressure in an overweight person.

Blood pressure can vary widely during a single day's time and can become elevated at a moment of stress. Such stress can result from a person's visit to a doctor's office to have his or her pressure taken. For this reason some physicians find it best to have a patient obtain a sphygmomanometer for measuring and recording his or her own blood pressure at home during specified periods.

EQUIPMENT AND NONDRUG SUPPLIES

Your doctor may recommend that you use certain kinds of diagnostic or health-related equipment or that you monitor your condition periodically. By taking your own blood pressure or testing your blood glucose level, for instance, you can avoid more frequent trips to the doctor's office. You can also treat some conditions yourself at home with heat lamps, wraps, and pads or with physical therapy equipment.

Blood Pressure Gauges

Your physician may ask you to take your own blood pressure at home on a regular basis and keep a record of your readings for his or her later review. There are two very good reasons for doing this: (1) the doctor may want to know how you are reacting at various times of the day and under differing conditions as an aid to prescribing treatment for your hypertension, and (2) the doctor may want you to see for yourself exactly what progress you are making toward controlling your high blood pressure. Because hypertension sometimes reveals few, if any, symptoms, some patients may reduce the frequency or amount of their medication or relax their observance of the doctor's dietary and activity warnings under the mistaken impression that their condition has improved. The use of a blood pressure measuring device (sphygmomanometer) is the only way a doctor—or you—can tell positively whether you are responding favorably to treatment.

Most people are familiar with the type of blood pressure cuff that utilizes either a column of mercury or a small round gauge to indicate pressure. This kind of cuff is used with a stethoscope for listening to the heartbeat as air is slowly released from the inflated cuff. For some persons it may be difficult to place the stethoscope properly under the cuff or to hear the heartbeat clearly. It may also be too cumbersome a procedure for the patient to handle alone.

There are new, battery-operated blood pressure devices on the market that do not require the use of a stethoscope and can be used easily by someone taking his or her own pressure reading. They still require the use of a cuff containing an inflatable bladder, but it is no longer necessary to listen for the heartbeat. Some of the devices include a large, illuminated, readable digital display of both the systolic and diastolic pressures as well as the heart rate. Others not only show a digital readout, but also have a printing feature that provides a permanent paper copy of the blood pressure, pulse rate, and date and time of each reading.

In order to monitor your blood pressure, it is necessary for you to be instructed in the proper technique by your physician or another health-care provider. Your pharmacist may also offer buying and operating tips. A simple anatomy lesson (so that you can easily locate the artery in your arm for correct positioning of a stethoscope) and instructions about what to listen for should be enough. If you decide to use one of the newer kinds of monitoring devices, ask your pharmacist for assistance in its use but also take it along with you on your next visit to the doctor's office for further instructions.

What Is Hypertension?

The word *hypertension* comes from two words meaning "overly tight" or "rigid." This does not mean that the person with hypertension is overly tight or rigid; it means that the person's blood vessels become tight and rigid for various reasons. The condition itself is usually caused by a narrowing of the peripheral blood vessels, that is, those that are relatively small and located farthest away from the heart, primarily in the arms and legs. Narrowing and constriction occur when deposits form on the inner walls of the vessels or when they lose some of their normal elasticity and become somewhat stiffer. When this happens, the heart has to pump a little harder in order to keep the blood circulating throughout the entire body.

It is often difficult, if not impossible, to determine the exact cause of an individual's hypertension. It could be the result of a narrowing within the body's principal artery, thyroid disease, an adrenal gland tumor, kidney disease, or any one of several other disturbances. It can also be caused by excessive mental strain and distress.

The symptoms of hypertension include throbbing headaches, unusual and excessive sweating, tingling in the limbs, a general feeling of uneasiness and apprehension, a pounding heartbeat, flushing of the face, and nausea and vomiting. However, it is also possible that a person can become hypertensive and show no outward signs of the disease. For this reason, hypertension is sometimes called the "silent killer."

continued on next page

A person is generally considered to be somewhat hypertensive—and it is important to remember that there are degrees of the disease—if his or her blood pressure registers over 140 systolic or 90 diastolic. Current estimates of the number of Americans suffering from hypertension range as high as 25 percent of the adult population. Because of the absence of overt symptoms, millions do not even suspect they have the disease. Those persons most likely to develop hypertension can generally, but not exclusively, be identified as belonging to certain groups: blacks with high blood pressure outnumber whites by three or four to one; smokers; those who drink more than moderate amounts of alcohol; those who favor heavily salted foods; those who are overweight; persons who are under unusual stress. Coronary artery disease, kidney failure, and stroke can result from a hypertensive condition.

Hypertension can generally be controlled by medication and careful monitoring of all contributing factors by both the patient and the doctor.

Glucose Monitoring

Diabetes self-management requires periodic testing of blood glucose levels, that is, the amount of unused sugar in the blood. Until recent years, diabetics had to rely on urine tests, which were often unreliable and inaccurate. Most self-monitoring now, however, is done by testing the blood itself, a far more dependable indicator of elevated sugar levels.

There are basically two kinds of testing procedures. Each involves puncturing a finger with a tiny lancet and allowing a drop of blood to flow onto a small, chemically coated test strip. With one method the strip is then matched against a color key in much the same way as earlier urine testing was done; the other method involves inserting the strip into a battery-powered device that reads the strip and displays the blood sugar value digitally. Your physician may express a preference for one or the other method; cost is a factor as well because the battery-operated reader is considerably more expensive. Make certain that you understand exactly how and when you are supposed to test your blood-sugar level. Ask your physician for precise instructions, do the test at least once in his or her office, and ask your pharmacist for instructions once again when you go to the drugstore to buy supplies.

One word of warning: if you are still relying on a urine test that includes the use of tablets, never store the bottle of tablets near any medications. They contain caustic soda and are poisonous when taken internally. Don't take the chance of mistaking them for some of your pills.

Heating Pads and Heat Lamps

Some people find heating pads to be effective for treating the pain associated with arthritis or muscle strain. A variety of electric heating pads or wraps is available, some of which provide either moist or dry heat. Some also have built-in vibrators designed to increase blood flow. (Caution: check with your doctor before using any appliance that vibrates, including foot-soak tubs, backrests, or chairs. Vibration could be hazardous, particularly for those persons who may be likely to produce blood clots.)

Heating pads should always be covered with a thick towel when in use and should never be used by anyone who is unconscious, unable to move, or sleeping. Never slide a heating pad under a bed patient; always apply the pad over the affected area. Burns and blistering can occur very quickly and can be quite severe.

Heat lamps can be effective for muscle aches, but the time under the lamp should be carefully monitored according to your physician's directions. Never leave an elderly or bedridden patient alone with a heat lamp burning over him or her. The lamps become very hot and can easily burn the person if left on too long.

Vaporizers

Vaporizers supply either hot or cold moist air by blowing out tiny droplets of water into a room. Since it is the moisturizing effect that is important, select a vaporizer that does not heat the water; it is safer. Moist air is effective for relieving congestion resulting from colds and will do as good a job as an OTC decongestant. Vaporizers should be kept scrupulously clean, because fungi and molds tend to accumulate in them. This may cause breathing problems when these organisms are released into the air by the vaporizer.

Incontinence Aids

Incontinence, not uncommon in the older patient, is more easily managed with the use of convenient products now available at full-service drugstores. There are not only waterproof sheets to protect beds and bedding, but also kits containing creams and ointments specifically formulated to relieve skin irritation resulting from prolonged exposure to urine. Specially designed briefs fitted with moistureproof shields and pads allow the incontinent person to leave home without fear of embarrassment. Discuss your need with your pharmacist and ask for guidance in making a selection of appropriate products.

Bathroom Appliances

Many larger drugstores now carry plastic leg and arm covers, made with nonadhesive fasteners, that make it possible for you to bathe without fear of dampening casts or dressings. They are reusable and are also suitable as coverings over hot packs.

For those persons who prefer to take a shower instead of a bath but are somewhat unsteady, there are small, portable benches made of noncorroding plastic and aluminum that can be placed inside a tub or shower stall, permitting them to remain seated while showering. Bathtubs can be fitted with detachable, but sturdy, handrails that offer firm support when climbing into and out of the tub.

3

HOW DRUGS WORK

Every medication has its own use or uses—what is called in the medical and pharmaceutical industries its *indications*. Prescription drugs can be categorized into several groups based on the drugs' use(s) and the therapeutic effect each drug has on certain systems in the body. Although each drug is intended to treat a certain condition and affect a certain body system, occasionally a drug will prove to have additional effects other than those intended. These may be side effects or an allergic reaction to the medication or even an interaction with food or another drug. In these cases, your doctor will have to judge whether you can continue to use the drug. In general, however, most prescription medicines will fall into one of the following classifications. Examples of drug families or types that are profiled in Part II of this book are marked with an asterisk.

DRUGS FOR THE CIRCULATORY SYSTEM

Drug therapy to treat disorders of the circulatory system has changed radically in the last 10 years. With the development of beta blockers and calcium channel blockers, treatment of heart and circulatory problems has been revolutionized. This, along with outstanding advances in surgical techniques and in technology, has reduced the death rate from heart disease and stroke by more than 25 percent since 1970.

Beta Blockers

Beta blockers are a group of drugs that block what are called *beta effects* produced by the adrenal hormones, adrenaline and noradrenaline. These two hormones can affect the heart, blood vessels, and lung passages by increasing the heart rate and the strength of the heart's contractions and by enlarging blood vessels. Beta blockers are used to block the beta effects in those conditions in which a stimulant effect is harmful. Because their blocking action decreases stimulation to the heart, the work of the heart is decreased. Therefore, these drugs are used to treat heartbeat irregularities (arrhythmias) and angina (chest pains caused by a diminished blood flow to the heart). They have also been found effective in reducing the number of second heart attacks. In addition, beta blockers are used to manage high blood pressure, either by decreasing heart output or by interfering with the release of renin, a hormone produced by the kidney that plays a part in contracting blood vessels and raising blood pressure. And finally, because these drugs block the enlargement of blood vessels, one of them has been approved for treating vascular headaches, such as migraine. It is thought that migraine headaches result from enlargement of the blood vessels in the scalp and/or changes in the blood vessels in the brain and neck.

Beta blockers are powerful drugs and may have side effects.

However, in most cases the benefits of their use far outweigh the problems. One of the more serious problems affects persons with asthma or other respiratory problems. The beta effects on the lungs cause the breathing passages to expand. If these effects are blocked, the breathing tubes may constrict and cause problems for people with respiratory conditions. However, there is a category of beta blockers that is referred to as being *cardioselective*. These drugs exert the desired effect on the heart but do not affect the lungs as much. Thus, under very special conditions and with medical supervision, they may be used by persons with certain respiratory conditions, although as a rule they should not be used by persons with asthma.

In addition, beta blockers may interfere with the blood sugar balance in diabetics who take insulin. Beta blockers can prevent the body from producing new sugar in the liver to counteract a state of low blood sugar caused by too much insulin intake. A diabetic can use a beta blocker only under very carefully controlled circumstances.

Beta blockers should not be discontinued abruptly because doing so causes a "rebound" effect in the body. In other words, stopping the drug without tapering off results in an extreme increase in blood pressure, angina pain, or whatever the beta blocker is being used to treat for. (Examples of beta blockers: Corgard*, Inderal*, Lopressor*, Tenormin*.)

Calcium Channel Blockers

Another recently developed group of drugs, calcium channel blockers interfere with the action of calcium in blood vessel walls. The result is that the drug relaxes the muscle in the walls of the blood vessels, improving the flow of blood. Calcium channel blockers also prevent spasms in these blood vessels and may, in some cases, relax the heart muscle, causing it to use less oxygen. These drugs are useful in the treatment of angina and high blood pressure. (Example of calcium channel blocker: Procardia*.)

High Blood Pressure Medications

As mentioned above, beta blockers and calcium channel blockers are used to treat high blood pressure. There are also other medications to manage this circulatory problem.

One of the main drug families used to treat high blood pressure is the diuretic group. In fact, diuretics alone can control high blood pressure in more than 40 percent of those persons afflicted. Diuretics cause the elimination of fluid and salt from the body. This reduces the actual fluid volume of the blood, which, in turn, lowers blood pressure. The most commonly used diuretics are the thiazide diuretics. These medications are well tolerated and are usually effective for the entire day. However, they do have one drawback: when they promote increased fluid loss, they also promote sodium and potassium loss. The sodium loss is desirable since sodium encourages fluid retention, but potassium depletion is not desirable and can even be detrimental. This can be compensated for by taking a potassium supplement (potassium chloride*) along with the diuretic. The pharmaceutical industry has also developed another type of diuretic that is called *potassium-sparing*. These diuretics have been combined with thiazide diuretics for the most effective antihypertensive action with the least loss of potassium. These medications are very commonly used. (Example of a potassium-sparing diuretic: Dyazide*.)

Another family of diuretics, called *loop diuretics*, are very powerful and very effective. However, as they cause more water loss, they also cause more potassium loss. (Example of a loop diuretic: Lasix*.)

There are medications in addition to beta blockers, calcium channel blockers, and diuretics that are prescribed to manage high blood pressure. Some work by dilating the blood vessels, thus decreasing the resistance within the vessels. Others act on the central nervous system to reduce heart output, heart rate, and resistance in the blood vessels. These drugs may be used alone or in combination with other blood pressure medications. (Examples of high blood pressure drugs: Aldomet*, Catapres*, Minipress*.)

Anti-Arrhythmic Drugs

If the heartbeat is not rhythmic or smooth, an anti-arrhythmic drug may be prescribed to restore the proper heartbeat. Quite often a beta blocker is used to block the stimulation causing the arrhythmia. If a person cannot take a beta blocker because of a prohibiting condition, there are other drugs that will correct an irregular heartbeat. (Example of an anti-arrhythmic: quinidine sulfate.)

Drugs Derived from Digitalis

These drugs are prescribed to regulate an irregular heartbeat, although they are not considered to be anti-arrhythmics. This group of medications slows down the heart rate but increases the strength of the contractions. Therefore, in addition to restoring a normal heartbeat, these medications may be used to stimulate increased output in heart failure. (Example of a digitalis-derived drug: Lanoxin*.)

Anti-Angina Drugs

If there is an insufficient supply of blood, and therefore of oxygen, to the heart, chest pain known as *angina* pain occurs. Drugs to relieve the pain cause an increased amount of oxygen to enter the heart. Nitroglycerine is the old standby to relieve angina pain, although beta blockers and calcium channel blockers are now also prescribed. (Examples of anti-angina drugs: Isordil*, nitroglycerin*.)

Anticoagulants

Anticoagulants, often commonly called *blood thinners*, prevent blood clotting. These drugs are prescribed for conditions such as abnormal blood clotting, stroke, and some forms of heart disease. Oral anticoagulants are derived from a compound called *warfarin* and are powerful drugs. Anyone taking an anticoagulant should be careful not to use other drugs, including aspirin, without consulting a doctor. In addition, if you are taking an oral anticoagulant, try to avoid any activity that may cause injury or bleeding, and take care in brushing your teeth and shaving so as not to induce bleeding. (Example of an anticoagulant: Coumadin★.)

DRUGS FOR THE DIGESTIVE SYSTEM

Although the most commonly prescribed drugs for the digestive system are those that are used to treat ulcers, there are other drugs available to manage other conditions of the gastrointestinal tract.

Ulcer Medications

There are two types of ulcer medications. One acts by inhibiting the secretion of stomach acid. The drugs Tagamet★ and Zantac★ work in this manner. Another type of drug forms a chemical barrier over the ulcer. Carafate works in this way. The purpose of both types of drugs is to relieve ulcer symptoms while promoting healing of the ulcer.

Drugs for Nausea and Diarrhea

Nausea drugs decrease the feeling of nausea and reduce the urge to vomit. There are powerful antinausea drugs that can be used for severe cases of nausea and vomiting. Compazine, a phenothiazine derivative, is an example of this kind of medication. More commonly used are antihistamines to prevent and reduce nausea. Dramamine★ is a drug that falls into this category.

If diarrhea cannot be controlled by a change in diet, some doctors may prescribe a narcotic or anticholinergic. A cholinergic action increases the intestine's peristalisis—the alternate contraction and relaxation of the bowel that propels food through. Thus an anticholinergic drug will block that kind of action and slow the action of the bowel. A narcotic drug works in the same way. Sometimes a combination of a narcotic and an anticholinergic drug is used. (Example of an antidiarrhea drug: Lomotil.)

DRUGS FOR THE RESPIRATORY SYSTEM

Several types of drugs are available for treating various respiratory ailments.

Bronchodilators

The word *bronchodilator* defines itself: this type of drug dilates, or enlarges, the bronchi, or breathing passages, in the lungs. These drugs are used by persons with asthma, emphysema, respiratory allergies, or chronic bronchitis. (Examples of bronchodilators: theophylline*, Ventolin*.)

Antihistamines

Antihistamines relieve the symptoms of an allergy by inhibiting the effects of histamine, a chemical released by the body when the person comes into contact with an allergen (the offending substance to which the person is allergic). Because some antihistamines may cause a person to feel drowsy, these drugs are sometimes the basis of sleeping medications. (Examples of antihistamines; Dimetane*, Seldane*.)

Decongestants

Decongestants open up airways in the nose and sinuses by constricting blood vessels in those areas. Because of the way in which they work, decongestants can raise blood pressure. You can use either oral or nasal decongestants. Oral medications are slow-acting, whereas applying a nasal decongestant, in the form of a spray or drops, brings almost immediate relief. In addition, sprays or drops do not raise the blood pressure as much as oral preparations. However, both forms can have what is known as the *rebound effect*. That is to say that while the medicine acts effectively for a period of time by constricting the blood vessels within the nasal passages, thus expanding the airway, eventually the walls of the vessels tire and begin to relax even beyond their normal state. After about three days the result can be greater congestion than before you began using the medication. Therefore, most doctors recommend that you do not use a decongestant for more than three days. (Examples of decongestants: Afrin*, Neo-Synephrine*, Sudafed*.)

Some doctors recommend combination products, made up

of a decongestant and an antihistamine. Others, however, feel that a single-ingredient preparation is better because that way you are avoiding unnecessary medications. Talk to your doctor before purchasing any of these products. (Example of combination products: Dimetapp*.)

Cough Medicines

There are two types of medications used for coughing: suppressants and expectorants. Cough suppressants reduce the frequency of the cough by suppressing the cough reflex in the cough center of the brain. They may be narcotic (codeine*) or nonnarcotic (Benylin*). Both are effective in treating a cough, but a narcotic may have a sedative effect.

Cough expectorants are supposed to change a nonproductive—dry and hacking—cough into a productive one, that is, one that brings up more phlegm. Few expectorants have been shown to be effective. Using a vaporizer or humidifier or even drinking water will probably be as effective as an expectorant.

Before deciding to use a cough medicine, remember that coughing is a defense mechanism, the body's method of removing irritating or harmful matter that enters the breathing system. A cough is as serious as the condition that is causing it. To eliminate the cough, it is best to eliminate the disease or condition that is setting off the coughing. While you are treating the underlying condition, you may want to allow the defense mechanism to work and not try to suppress the cough. On the other hand, if the coughing is so severe that you cannot sleep, you may decide to use a cough suppressant, especially at night. (Example of an expectorant: Robitussin*.)

DRUGS FOR THE NERVOUS SYSTEM

You may be surprised to find some of these drugs listed as working on the nervous system. For example, the painkiller you take for arthritis does not act on the arthritis but on the nervous system, to kill the pain. Other drugs, such as sedatives and tranquilizers, are more obvious as nervous system drugs.

Painkillers

Painkillers do not cure, but rather relieve, a symptom. Although relieving pain is important, obtaining pain relief without attempting to discover or eliminate the underlying cause of the pain may be dangerous. On the other hand, some conditions, such as arthritis, perhaps cannot be eliminated. In these cases pain relief is the primary goal.

Painkillers can be narcotic or nonnarcotic. Narcotic painkillers act on the brain, producing pain relief and a sense of well-being. However, they can be addictive. (Example of a narcotic painkiller: codeine★.)

Nonnarcotic painkillers are more commonly used, and they are not addictive. The best known, of course, is aspirin. An aspirin substitute, acetaminophen, is also commonly used, although it does not relieve inflammation and therefore is not recommended for arthritis patients. There are also prescription painkillers for more serious conditions. (Examples of prescription painkillers: Darvocet-N★, Fiorinal★.)

Another effective painkiller is a combination drug, consisting of narcotic and nonnarcotic ingredients. Tylenol with Codeine★ is one such combination product.

Again, because there is a narcotic ingredient in these products, a drug dependence problem can develop.

Anti-Inflammatory Drugs

Anti-inflammatory drugs are often considered a separate category even though one of their actions is to kill pain. Aspirin is the most commonly used antiinflammatory. Steroid drugs (see "Drugs for the Hormonal System," below) also fight inflammation. And there is a separate subclassification of anti-inflammatories: nonsteriod anti-inflammatory drugs (NSAID). (Examples of NSAID: Clinoril★, Feldene★, Indocin★, Naprosyn★, Nuprin★.)

Sedatives

Sedatives are used to treat anxiety and insomnia. They all work by decreasing activity in the brain. Both the drugs used to combat anxiety and those used to induce sleep act in the same manner, but the sleep-inducing drugs, also called *hypnotics*, are more potent. (Examples of sedatives with calming effect: Tranxene★, Valium★. Example of sleep-inducing sedatives: Dalmane★.)

Tranquilizers

Tranquilizers work by exerting a calming effect on certain parts of the brain while allowing the rest of the brain to function normally. They act as a filter, allowing some impulses to be received and others to be banned. These medications are usually prescribed for persons with psychotic illnesses. Often these persons are also depressed. In such cases, antidepressants, which also fall within this drug category, may be recommended. (Example of tranquilizer: Thorazine.)

Anticonvulsants

Anticonvulsants are used to prevent and control the convulsions and symptoms of epilepsy. They work by decreasing stimulation to the brain in a selective fashion. (Examples of anticonvulsants: Dilantin★, phenobarbital★.)

DRUGS FOR THE HORMONAL SYSTEM

The hormonal system, also known as the *endocrine system*, is quite complex and influences a great many functions of the body. The endocrine system is composed of the body's glands: pitui-tary gland, thyroid and parathyroid glands, pancreas, adrenal glands, and sex glands. Each of these glands secretes it own hormones, chemical messengers that travel through the bloodstream to various parts of the body where they direct or stimulate body functions. If the body's glands do not produce enough hormones, hormone drugs may be prescribed to compensate for the lack of natural hormones.

Steroid Drugs

Steroids are naturally produced in the body by the adrenal glands after being stimulated by adrenocorticotropic hormone (ACTH), secreted by the pituitary gland. Steroids, whether in the natural or drug form, fight inflammation. Thus, steroids are often prescribed to relieve the symptoms of arthritis or other inflammatory diseases. (Example of a steroid drug: prednisone★.)

Thyroid Supplements

For the individual whose thyroid gland does not produce sufficient amounts of thyroid hormone, the development of thyroid supplements has been extremely important. Originally, thyroid supplements were manufactured by grinding up the dried thyroid glands of animals and forming them into tablets. Now, however, a synthetic thyroid hormone supplement (Synthroid★) is also available.

Antidiabetes Drugs

Insulin, a hormone secreted by the pancreas, controls the body's use of glucose, or sugar, by carrying the glucose to the cells for energy or to the liver for storage until needed for energy. If the pancreas does not produce enough insulin or if the body cannot use the insulin produced by the pancreas, diabetes is the result.

Fortunately, insulin★ replacement is available. For many years insulin has been derived from animal pancreases, but now human insulin is available. It is not taken from human beings but is manufactured in a synthetic process. Insulin is injected because, if taken orally, it would be digested before it accomplished its purpose.

Oral antidiabetes drugs are also available, but only for those persons who do not need insulin or who cannot control their diabetes by diet. These drugs stimulate the pancreas to produce more insulin. However, oral antidiabetes medications cannot be used by diabetics whose pancreases do not produce insulin; only insulin injections will be prescribed for these people. (Example of an oral antidiabetic: Diabinese★.)

Sex Hormones

Sex hormones are secreted primarily by the sex glands, called *ovaries* in a woman and *testes* in a man. The female hormones, estrogen and progesterone, develop and maintain the female sex characteristics, such as breast development, menstrual cycle, preparation of the uterus for pregnancy, and other feminine physical traits. The male sex hormone is testosterone, and its function is to develop and maintain the male sex characteristics, such as sperm production, beard, increased muscle mass, and deepened voice.

Sex hormone supplements are most often used by women over 50 years old who are experiencing menopausal symptoms related directly to reduced secretion of the sex hormones. At one time estrogen replacement was the primary treatment for postmenopausal women to prevent the hot flashes and vaginal dryness that may accompany menopause. Then research showed that estrogen replacement also helped to guard against osteoporosis, a thinning of the bones. However, taking estrogen after menopause was found to increase the risk of endometrial cancer—cancer of the lining of the uterus. Now, however, research has shown that taking estrogen along with progesterone replacements reduces the risk of endometrial cancer; in essence, the replacement hormones are mimicking the natural hormonal balance during premenopause years. Thus, women and their doctors are reconsidering hormonal replacement therapy. This is not to say that every woman can or should take hormone supplements; in fact, some women definitely should not take these medications. Discuss with your doctor whether or not you need or are eligible for this kind of therapy. Premarin* is a female hormone (estrogen) supplement that may be used with Provera, a progesterone supplement.

DRUGS FOR THE EYES

There are three basic types of eye medications: antibiotic, steroid, and glaucoma medication. Antibiotic eye drops are used to treat infections, and steroids may be used for inflammation. Steroid eye drops are safe if used for a short period of time. However, most pharmacists will not refill a prescription for steroid eye drops without approval from the prescribing doctor.

Glaucoma medication is prescribed to reduce the increased pressure within the eyeball that is the main characteristic of glaucoma. Timoptic* is such a drug. Timoptic's ingredient is a beta blocking drug (see above), and although it is not known exactly how Timoptic works, it is thought that it acts to reduce fluid formation within the eye as well as to promote fluid drainage. Use of this and similar drugs can prevent blindness that may occur if glaucoma is not treated.

DRUGS TO FIGHT INFECTIONS

Several categories of medications fall into this group, and each one fights a specific type of infection.

Antibiotics

Antibiotics fight bacterial infections but are not effective against viruses. That is why antibiotics should not be prescribed for the common cold, which can be caused by any one of many viruses, although any of these viruses can lower your resistance to a bacterial infection for which an antibiotic may be prescribed. Antibiotics work by destroying the bacteria causing the infection. These medications are generally quite effective when taken as prescribed. However, many people stop taking the medication prematurely, that is, as soon as they begin to feel better. This may allow a reinfection to develop. (Examples of antibiotics: amoxicillin*, Augmentin*, Ceclor*, erythromycin*, Keflex*, penicillin V*, tetracycline*.)

Other Infection Fighters

There are drugs to combat other infections that are not caused by bacteria. For example, there are drugs that prevent and destroy fungus infections (Mycostatin*). Antiviral medications are prescribed to treat virus infections. Sulfa drugs treat certain infections, such as urinary tract infections and certain types of ear and respiratory infections (Bactrim*, Gantrisin*). And finally there are drugs that treat worm, lice, and scabies infestations. Lindane* is commonly used to eliminate lice, for example.

4

BUYING OVER-THE-COUNTER PRODUCTS

A recent FDA study estimates that about two-thirds of the ingredients contained in OTC products are ineffective or at least merit further study in order to determine precisely how effective they might be. A few ingredients are actually harmful. This means that only approximately one-third of OTC product ingredients have actually been proven to be effective. This is not to say, of course, that there are no good nonprescription medications. There are, as a matter of fact, many products that you can buy without a doctor's order that are very helpful and are essential parts of personal good health care and preventive medicine.

When you consider that there are now more than a quarter of a million patent medicines, remedies, tonics, elixirs, pills, salves, lotions, capsules, and powders on the market, the problem of determining whether the medication you purchase is really going to help you can become staggering. How can you find out whether the drug you are using is any good?

No layperson can be expected to evaluate every kind of product sold at the corner drugstore. It therefore becomes necessary to turn to a professional for help in selecting a medication that will treat your complaint effectively, inexpensively, and safely. The best source of that information is your pharmacist. He or she is an expert in determining precisely which one of a possibly staggering variety of products will do the job you want done. Just as physicians have been trained to treat illnesses by prescribing specific medicines, pharmacists have been trained in the chemical makeup of those medicines. They know how drugs are formulated, which drugs may react with other substances, and how drugs should be stored and administered.

Your pharmacist is a good source of information about the

effectiveness of a particular medication, its cost, and the best way to take the medicine to prevent additional discomfort or the possibility of a troublesome reaction. Since there may be a generic version of the product that contains the same ingredients and costs far less than a popularly advertised brand-name item, it is always best to discuss price with your pharmacist. It costs a lot of money for large pharmaceutical manufacturers to advertise their products on radio and television and in newspapers and magazines, and that expense is passed along to you, the consumer, in the price of the products. Generic versions of the same products ride along on the coattails of heavily advertised items and usually cost much less. Of course, generic equivalents do not exist for every one of the many OTC medicines, but you can realize considerable savings on those that are available.

Do not assume that simply because a product is stocked in your favorite drugstore it is worthwhile to purchase. As noted above, some OTC medications may not perform specifically as their advertising implies, nor may they be at all necessary for treating minor ailments. The druggist oftentimes has little or no control over the variety of products stocked in his or her store, espe-

cially if he or she is a staff pharmacist employed by a chain of stores.

When purchasing OTC medications, always try to find a single-ingredient product that will treat your specific complaint. That may be difficult to do because many medicines are compounds of several ingredients designed to treat as broad a range of symptoms as possible, thus making them more widely saleable. Again, your pharmacist may be able to recommend a product for you that contains no ingredients other than those required to relieve the symptoms you are suffering. Even those products that contain only a single medically active ingredient often contain preservatives or fillers. By selecting single-ingredient products you are able to treat only your specific symptoms and thus avoid taking other chemicals into your body that you do not need.

Because of the prevalence of multiple ingredients in OTC medications, it is necessary for you to become a careful reader of labels. If the print is too small for you to read easily, or if some of the ingredients listed are chemical names that are unfamiliar to you, ask the druggist for assistance in determining whether a particular product is the right one for you. Some of the extra ingredients can cause you to experience an adverse reaction, especially if you are taking certain prescription medications at the same time.

SELECTING A PHARMACY

Chances are you have been patronizing the same drugstore for a number of years or at least have done most of your buying at two or three stores that you have found to be convenient. If you are now in the position of being a fairly frequent buyer of either prescription or nonprescription medicines, it is best to confine your shopping to one store where you can get to know the staff—especially the pharmacist—and where they know you. Choosing a pharmacy is in some respects like choosing a physican. You need to find someone you can trust who will take the time to talk to you and explain how the medicines you buy work, react, and interact.

If you have been in the habit of picking up pain remedies and cough syrup at the grocery or convenience store and have not had occasion to buy prescriptions, make the change now. Continue to buy your toiletries and notions wherever it is handiest for you, but save your medical purchases for the drugstore where there is a trained and registered pharmacist on duty at all times.

Ask the druggist for advice and suggestions even if you are not having a prescription filled. Ask whether the antacid you have been using for the past 10 years is really the best one for you. Explain any kinds of aches, pains, and cold discomforts you occasionally have and ask how you might best treat them. Ask about new brands of first aid supplies or household health gadgets and how they work. In short, talk to the pharmacist and get to know him or her.

The time may come when you need to have a question answered about whether it is wise to take a particular OTC remedy while also taking a drug your doctor has prescribed. The druggist will be more receptive and willing to offer an explanation if he or she already knows you and is accustomed to your inquiries and routine purchases.

Select a drugstore that is convenient, one that you can make "your" drugstore. It may be a small, independently owned store, a large chain store in a shopping mall, or the drug department in a department store. The larger stores may have two or three pharmacists on duty during different shifts if they are open for long hours, and they may rotate their professional staffs among several stores. Obviously, it is considerably more difficult to get to know specific pharmacists in that kind of situation, and for that reason you may choose to patronize another store, one with a more settled pharmacy department. Try to avoid stores where you simply hand a prescription to a counter assistant who then passes it back to an unseen pharmacist. The whole point of carefully selecting a drugstore is to find one with an accessible pharmacist who can give you sound professional advice. You won't get that if you can't talk directly to the pharmacist.

Several factors should be considered when choosing a pharmacy:

• Check the pharmacy's hours. If it is in a large store, is the pharmacy department open the same hours as the rest of the store? Is it open on Sundays? Does it provide after-hours emergency service?
• Does the pharmacy offer a delivery service in case you are unable to get in?
• Is it convenient to your home? If you must take public transportation to get there, is that transportation available on weekends?
• Does it carry a wide selection of products, including generic or private-label items that may be less expensive than well-known brand items?

• Are its prices competitive? Does the store offer a senior citizen discount? Will it accept Medicare and Medicaid customers?
• Does it offer credit or accept major bank credit cards? (This latter point could be important if you expect to have a friend or neighbor pick up your order for you.)
• If it is part of a large chain, does your local store have a computer capability that will enable it to forward your records to other stores in the chain so that you can make your prescription purchases elsewhere if more convenient? Will the pharmacist enter into the computer all the drugs you are using so that a possible interaction can be anticipated and prevented?
• Most importantly, is the pharmacist courteous, friendly, and, above all, helpful?

CHOOSING OTC PRODUCTS

Most patent medicines are intended to provide relief from the symptoms of common illnesses and the discomfort associated with temporary or lasting non-acute complaints and conditions; they are rarely meant to be cures for diseases. Serious or potentially serious diseases caused by bacterial or viral infections generally require professional attention and strong medication that will kill the invading organisms and can be ordered only by a physician. Some of the symptoms of even those ailments can, however, often be alleviated by nonprescription drugs.

Knowing which medicines to select from among the many available may be difficult without some kind of guidance. Your pharmacist is the best source of that kind of helpful information. Explain the kinds of symptoms you are experiencing, how long you have had them, and what, if anything, you have already been doing for relief. Be certain to tell the pharmacist—don't wait to be asked—if you have high blood pressure, diabetes, or heart disease or if you suffer frequent stomach upset. It is very important that you volunteer this information because some OTC medications contain ingredients that, although safe for the population in general, may be irritating or harmful to someone with a preexisting illness or condition. If you are taking any other kind of medicine—whether it is a prescription or another kind of patent remedy—you must be certain to tell the pharmacist. Some OTC medicines—even such common ones as aspirin, cold remedies, and antacids—can react with some prescription drugs and change their effectiveness. Also, if you are using another kind of OTC medicine, the ingredients in the one recommended by your pharmacist may be similar to what you are already taking, and you could be risking an overdose.

The ingredients in OTC drugs, just as those in prescription medicines, are potentially powerful, and they can react with other chemicals contained in certain foods, beverages, or other medicines. Keep in mind that medicines that are given orally can react with other medicines that are used topically, that is, applied externally. Ask the pharmacist about the possibility of side effects from taking his or her recommended OTC medication. Are there some minor reactions that you should expect? What would a serious reaction be, and how would you recognize it? What kind of reaction would be dangerous enough to call your doctor about? (In the event you experience a serious reaction from any kind of drug, prescription or OTC, do not call your pharmacist. Call your doctor. Tell the doctor exactly what you are feeling and what you have taken.)

Finally, ask the pharmacist if the product you have selected is the most economical yet effective way to treat your ailment. Your pharmacist can help you save money by suggesting alternative products that may be cheaper or by vouching for the safety and effectiveness of a lower-priced generic or store-brand product. In general, this latter point applies only when you are treating an ailment yourself; if your physician recommends or prescribes a particular item by brand name, you should follow his or her advice.

Reading the Label

Before buying any product, read the label carefully. The label should include this information:

- the name and type of drug
- its purpose
- dosage
- the maximum safe dosage
- instructions for the drug's use
- directions for storing the drug
- warnings, including possible side effects, drug interactions, and special health problems that might interfere with the use of the drug
- the drug's active ingredients (manufacturers are not required to specify concentrations or strengths of ingredients for some products; if the concentrations are not listed, don't buy the product)

- expiration date (the date beyond which the drug should not be used for the sake of safety or effectiveness)
- the name and address of the manufacturer

If all of this information is not on the label, do not buy the drug. Even if your pharmacist is able to fill in the missing information for you, you may not remember it a month later if you have to use the medicine again. If the information is present but confusing, talk to the pharmacist and ask for clarification. Always be certain you know exactly what a drug will or will not do and how it should be used.

TAKING OTC MEDICINES

The importance of using an OTC medicine exactly the way the manufacturer suggests cannot be overemphasized. Extensive research and testing go into health-care products before they reach the market, and it is only reasonable to heed the advice of the firm that has formulated and tested the product.

Even after you have read the label in the drugstore and perhaps asked the druggist to clarify any unclear information, read the label again after you get home and before you use the medication. It's a good idea, in fact, to reread the label each time you take any kind of medicine.

Remember, practically any substance, including very common and seemingly harmless products, can be harmful if used incorrectly. Just as with prescription medications, misuse of an OTC drug can render it at best ineffective and at worst dangerous.

5

BUYING PRESCRIPTION DRUGS

Have you ever gone to the doctor for a specific illness or complaint, been handed a prescription, accepted it without question, had it filled at the drugstore, taken the medicine, and never known exactly what it was, precisely what it was supposed to do, or how it worked? If you are like the majority of people, your answer is probably yes.

Doctors are busy people in whom we place an enormous amount of faith and trust. Many people hesitate to "take up the doctor's time with a bunch of questions," preferring instead to assume that they have been told all they really need to know and that "the doctor knows best." That's true to a point, but what if the doctor, who may very well be busy and hurried, overlooks telling you about a reaction that may likely occur when you take the drug he or she has prescribed? The reaction may be normal and expected—at least by the doctor—but it may come as a com-

plete, and worrisome, surprise to you. Could this sort of situation be avoided? Of course it could, and it's your responsibility to see that it is.

You and your physician are partners in your health care. Think of yourself as part of a team whose job it is to keep you in the best possible health. One of the important aspects of that job is becoming informed about your physical condition and how it is being managed. And the best way to become informed is to ask questions of everyone who has something to do with your treatment. That includes your doctor(s), nurses, pharmacist, and anyone else who is involved in helping you stay healthy.

Once you have left the doctor's office and the drugstore, you and you alone are responsible for how you use the medicine that has been prescribed for you. Remember that medicines are potent substances that you are putting into your body. The chemicals are supposed to be beneficial, of course, but every person reacts a little differently to them. You should understand how the drug works; what to expect in the way of side effects, if any; what side effects or reactions are minor and expected; and which ones warrant a prompt call to your doctor.

Doctors and pharmacists are professionally trained to know about drugs, but you are the one whose responsibility it is to take the medicine and to observe its effects. In that case, shouldn't you tap the professional expertise of your doctor and pharmacist before you begin taking the medication?

The first step in using a prescription occurs in your doctor's office when you are handed the prescription. This is the time to ask specific questions about the drug(s) so that you are certain about (1) what you are supposed to do and (2) what the drug is supposed to do. Ask about side effects and warning signs. Ask precisely how you should take the drug. Ask what you should expect to happen after you have taken it. Ask about its cost. This is the time to clarify any doubts or questions you may have. One of the best ways to do this is to have a list of questions ready to use as a checklist when you discuss a prescription drug with your physician.

Let's take a closer look at some of these questions. It is important to know the name of the medicines you are taking in case you experience a reaction to them and have to tell someone other than your doctor what has happened. Also, you might ask your doctor to indicate on the prescription form that the pharmacist is to fill the prescription with the least expensive compound. Keep in mind that some medicines your doctor prescribes may have generic or even OTC equivalents that cost less than a brand-name product.

When you ask the doctor precisely what the drug is supposed to do, also find out if the prescribed medicine will simply speed up the desired therapeutic process or if it is essential to a cure. In other words, is it likely that you may get over your present problem with no medicine at all, although it may take a little longer?

As you prepare to take the drug, are the instructions clear? For example, is the instruction "Give four times a day" the same as "Give every six hours"? In general, these two sets of instructions are not interchangeable. If the label tells you to take the medicine four times a day, that means you should take the four doses of medication at evenly spaced intervals throughout your

What to Ask the Doctor

Sometimes when you go to see your doctor, particularly at those times when you have had to be squeezed into the doctor's schedule on an emergency basis, he or she may not have much time to spend with you. Nevertheless, there are still questions to which you need answers regarding prescribed medications. You can save your time and the doctor's—and still get all the information you need—if you jot down these questions ahead of time and run through them quickly when you see your doctor.

- What is the medication's name—both brand name and generic name? (The generic name is usually the name of the ingredients.)
- What is the drug supposed to do?
- How should I take the medication?
- How much medicine should I take at each dose?
- How often should I take this medicine?
- Am I supposed to take this medicine on a regular schedule—such as every four hours—or should I take it as I need it? How will I know when or if I need it?
- If I am supposed to take this medicine every four hours, does that mean throughout the night or only during the day?
- Should I take this medicine with food or on an empty stomach? Should I drink any more water than usual?
- Are there any foods or beverages I should or should not consume while taking this drug?
- Will this drug interfere with any lab tests I may have?
- Are there any minor side effects that I should expect, and can I take care of them myself?
- Are there any adverse side effects that I should call you about?
- Will this drug interact with any other medicines, including over-the-counter remedies, that I am using?
- Could I be allergic to this drug?
- What should I do if I miss a dose?
- If I am supposed to take this drug for a prolonged period of time, does it have any cumulative effect?
- Finally, what is perhaps the most important question of all—and don't hesitate to ask it: Is this drug really necessary? Do the benefits outweigh the risks?

waking hours. However, "every six hours" means that you must be very precise and take the medicine every six hours around the clock. In this case, you may have to set an alarm clock in order not to miss any doses.

The reason for differing timing instructions is that different medicines require different periods of time to become effective. Some medications must be taken at precisely spaced intervals around the clock in order to provide constant benefits. Others can be effective when taken during your normal waking day. Be sure you understand when and how often you should take any drug prescribed for you.

FOLLOWING DIRECTIONS

It is important to know exactly how long you should continue taking any medicine. Should it be for a certain number of days or just until you begin feeling well again? Some medicines have both symptomatic relief properties and specific disease-curing functions. You could feel much better in a couple of days, and your doctor could still want you to continue taking the medicine. In cases of some bacterial infections, for example, it is necessary to continue the medication for at least 10 days in order to cure the condition, even though you may feel well after only three or four days. Stopping the medication too soon can cause a relapse or complications. Quite often, the symptoms disappear long before the healing process is completed. Therefore, if your prescription label instructs you to "take entire contents," "take for 10 full days," or "continue for two weeks," carry out this instruction to the letter. This type of medication has a bigger job than just relieving symptoms.

Also ask your doctor about taking the medication with or without food. Find out as well if you should avoid certain foods or drinks while taking this drug. For example, you should never drink any alcoholic beverages if you are taking any drug to help you sleep. On the other hand, sometimes foods can be beneficial when eaten with a medication. Yogurt, for instance, can help prevent the mild diarrhea that may be a side effect of some antibiotics. When an antibiotic is taken to kill bacteria causing, say, an earache, the drug kills other bacteria in the body as well. Some bacteria normally living in the intestines are beneficial, and if the medication kills them, diarrhea may be the result. Yogurt that has been cultured with beneficial bacteria may help restore the normal balance of the intestine and thus works to prevent the diarrhea.

Some medicines are to be taken on an "as needed" basis. But what does "as needed" mean? What should you look for before applying an ointment or cream? How will you know exactly when to take another pill? Get specific instructions so that you avoid overusing the drug but still treat the ailment or condition effectively.

Some medications, such as drugs for urinary tract infections, require the flushing effect of more than the usual amount of water passing through the kidneys. It is very important that you know whether the prescription your doctor writes involves such a medicine.

Check each of these points with your doctor before taking any medicine your doctor prescribes. It is just possible he or she may forget to inform you completely. Sometimes a physician may rely on a pharmacist to inform a patient fully, and the pharmacist may assume the physician has already done so. Make it your responsibility to find out.

If the doctor is going to order any blood, urine, or other kinds of tests, ask whether the prescribed medicine will have any effect on their results. It may be best to wait until after the tests before beginning to take the medicine.

YOUR RESPONSE TO DRUGS

You will probably notice some change in your condition once you have begun taking a recommended medication. Ideally, it will be a diminishment in the illness for which the medicine was prescribed. But some adverse reactions could also occur. Is it a normal side effect of the drug, for example, for you to become sleepy or develop a slightly dry throat or upset stomach? Are there more serious reactions you should be watching for, such as blurry vision or a tendency to bleed more than usual from a slight cut? Which side effects are transitory and expected, and which ones should alert you to call your doctor? Some drugs are very powerful chemicals; know what you are dealing with.

Some allergies seem to occur in groups. That is, when you are allergic to one substance, it may be assumed that you may also be sensitive to another. In general, your physician will not know what your allergies are unless you describe them; do not fail to do so before accepting any medicine prescription. And be certain to tell your doctor if you are taking any over-the-counter remedies. Keep in mind that many medicines are compounds of more than one substance. While you may not have a reaction to the primary drug, you could be allergic to one of the other ingredients in the compound. It is even possible to have a reaction to the substance used to coat a pill while having no reaction to the actual medicine the pill contains.

YOUR RESPONSIBILITY

Just as your physician has the duty to answer your questions, you have an equally important responsibility to tell the doctor everything that pertains to your health:

- Are you seeing and being treated by any other health-care professional(s), including other medical doctors, a chiropractor, podiatrist, etc.?
- Are you taking other prescription drugs, including others previously prescribed by the doctor you are now seeing?
- Do you use any OTC medicines on a regular basis?
- Are you allergic to anything, or do you feel that you may be sensitive to certain kinds of drugs?
- Are you on a special diet or taking vitamin and mineral supplements?

Your doctor needs to have this information so that he or she can prescribe safely and effectively. Don't hesitate to remind your doctor also of any drug or treatment he or she may have recommended; most doctors see a large number of patients and are unable to keep track of every one of them without referring to their charts. If your doctor is not reading your record at the moment the prescription is being written, he or she may not precisely remember earlier suggestions or treatment. It is helpful to take all of your medicines with you when you visit the doctor. Be forthright and frank about all of your health practices. Most especially, tell your doctor about any other doctor who is treating you and any other drugs you are taking. Incidentally, the converse is true: be certain to inform any other doctors, dentists, or medical specialists of what you are taking and what medical professionals are treating you. It's a good idea to give each medical professional the names and telephone numbers of all health-care providers you are seeing.

READING THE PRESCRIPTIONS

Many people regard doctors' prescriptions as one of the great mysteries of life. Actually, they aren't terribly difficult to understand once you learn what various abbreviations mean. Prescriptions are written in a kind of shorthand that is based in large part on Latin and Greek terms, a carryover from the days when formal education included study of those languages. Nowadays it is unlikely that most physicians or pharmacists could even tell you the precise foreign-language meanings of the abbreviations they use, but they continue to use them nonetheless. Chalk it up to the mystique of the medical professions, but don't let it intimidate you.

When you are handed a prescription form by your doctor, read it over. If there are any terms you are unable to understand, ask for an explanation. And don't be satisfied with a reassuring "Don't worry about it. It will help you. The drugstore will give you directions." Tell your doctor you want to know what the medicine is and you want to know exactly how to use it. Later on you can ask the pharmacist the same questions, not necessarily to check up on your doctor but to reinforce the pertinent information you need to know.

When you do have the prescription filled, it will not be possible for you to know whether the pharmacist has carried out your doctor's orders properly unless you can knowledgeably compare the medicine's label with what was written on the prescription form. Mistakes can happen; even something as simple as a typographical error—say, the substitution of a *2* for a *4*—can occur when the pharmacist types out the instruction label. Another common and very serious error is the misplacement of a decimal point. The result may be a medicine ten times more potent than intended. In addition to reading the prescription against the medicine container's label, check the color, shape, and size of the tablet or capsule; be certain they are the same when buying a refill. Generic drugs are usually a different size, shape, or color, but if they are purchased from the same pharmacy, the results should be constant. Pay attention to what your physician and pharmacist tell you and don't hesitate to ask questions anytime you fail to understand precisely what you are supposed to do and watch for.

BUYING THE PRESCRIBED DRUG

When you buy a prescription medication, talk to your pharmacist. Discuss any new or additional questions that you may have neglected to ask your physi-

Pharmaceutical Abbreviations

Abbreviation	Meaning	Full Term (Latin unless otherwise indicated)
a; aa	of each	ana (Greek)
a c	before meals	ante cibum
ad lib	as wanted	ad libitum
aq	water	aqua
bib	drink	bibe
bid	twice a day	bis in die
bin	twice a night	bis in noctus
C	centigrade	Centigradus
c	with	cum
cap(s)	capsule(s)	capsula
cc	cubic centimeter	(French)
cg	centigram	(French)
cm	centimeter	(French)
comp	compound	compositus
dil	dilute	dilue
dr	dram(s)	drachma
elix	elixir	(Arabic)
et	and	et
ext	extract	extractum
F	Fahrenheit	(proper name)
Fld	fluid	fluidus
ft	make (let there be made)	fiat
gm	gram	gramme (French)
gr	grain	granum
gtt	drops	guttae
H	hour	hora
h n	tonight	hac nocte
h s	at bedtime	hora somni
hypo	hypodermically	(Greek)
i; ii; iii	one; two; three	I; II; III (Roman numerals)
L	liter	litra

liq	liquid; fluid	liquor
mg	milligram	(French)
mist	mixture	mistura
ml	milliliter	(French)
no	number	numero
non rep	don't repeat (refill)	non repetatur
noxt	at night	nocte, noxte
os	mouth	os, ora
oz	ounce	uncia
p c	after meals	post cibum
per	by, through	per
pil(s)	pill(s)	pilula
p o	by mouth	per os
prn	as needed	pro re nata
pulv	powder	pulvis
q h	every hour	quaque hora
q2h	every two hours	——
q4h	every four hours	——
qid	four times a day	quater in die
q s	sufficient quantity	quantum sufficiat
quotid	every day	quotidie
q v	as much as desired	quantum vis
rep	repeat (refill)	repetatur
Rx	take	recipe
S	mark	signa
s	without	sine
Sig	label (directions)	signetur
sol	solution	solutio
solv	dissolve	solve
ss	half	semis
stat	immediately	statim
syr	syrup	syrups
T	temperature	temperatura
tab(s)	tablet(s)	tabella
tid	three times a day	ter in die
tin	three times a night	ter in nocte
tr; tinct	tincture	tinctura
ung	ointment	unguentum

Note: Any of these abbreviations may appear with or without periods. If your doctor uses abbreviations other than those above, ask what they mean.

cian. The pharmacist can also inform you about price and money-saving ideas. Although he or she may not know the treatment regimen your doctor has decided on, the pharmacist does know about drugs and can tell you about the product you are buying.

As mentioned earlier, it is also a good idea to buy all of your drugs from the same pharmacy. A good professional pharmacy maintains detailed records for each customer, and often the pharmacist is the first person to discover that a new prescription will interact with a drug the patient is already using. Even though you think you have told your doctor about any other drugs you are taking, you may have forgotten one. In addition, a pharmacist who is familiar with your records and your family will know how to suggest OTC products that will not interfere with any prescription drugs you are taking. Another reason for staying with the same pharmacy is that you may be able to avoid the variability of generic drugs. The strength of generic drugs may vary. However, if you go to the same pharmacist who buys his or her generic drugs from the same manufacturer, you will get a constant dose of medication. This can be very important if you and your doctor are in the process of adjusting your dosage for any number of reasons. It is impor-

tant to develop a good working relationship with a professional pharmacist.

You will note that the questions you should ask your pharmacist may often be the same ones you have asked your doctor. This is because the doctor and the pharmacist are approaching your illness from two different angles: the doctor is the expert on illness and treatment, and the pharmacist is the expert on the chemical makeup of medications. While your doctor and your pharmacist may give you much the same answers to your questions, the pharmacist might give you a little more information about the practical administration of drugs. It also doesn't hurt to ask the same questions twice so that you are absolutely certain that you know what to do. By the way, if you begin to experience an adverse reaction to a prescription medication, phone your physician at once; don't call the pharmacist. Don't rely on your pharmacist for treatment; that's the job of your doctor.

DRUG FRESHNESS AND STORAGE

Most OTC remedies have expiration dates printed on their labels. These are specific dates beyond which you should not use the medicine. Prescription drugs

What to Ask the Pharmacist

- What is the maximum amount of this medication that I should use in one day?
- How should this drug be stored?
- What is the expiration date for this medicine? How long will it be safe and effective?
- Is there an OTC product that is equally effective and perhaps less expensive?
- Is there a generic equivalent that is just as effective and cheaper?
- How many refills will be available?
- In your experience, what are the common side effects associated with this drug? When should I call my doctor about a side effect?
- How much of this medication should I buy at one time? (This question applies to a medication for a long-term condition; for an acute illness the doctor generally prescribes a limited amount of medication to handle the short-term condition.)
- Will this medication interact with any other prescription drugs or OTC medicines I am now taking?
- Is there anything else I should know about this medication?
- Is there a printed patient education brochure available for this medication, and, if so, may I have a copy?

generally carry no such time indications. All drugs age, whether they are prescription or nonprescription, and aging can alter the effectiveness of their ingredients. Most often aging will decrease the strength of the product, but there are many instances in which aging will actually cause the medicine to become toxic. Therefore, taking any medication that you have had on hand for a long period of time can be foolhardy because at best it may not perform according to your expectations; at worst it could cause a serious problem to develop.

As a general rule, medications of any kind should not be kept beyond one year after their purchase, whether or not they have an expiration date on the label. Opening a sealed container and allowing air to reach the contents can begin an immediate deterioration of the active ingredients. Tablets, capsules, liquids, and ointments age at different rates, and some medications are more affected than others by heat, light, or moisture.

While prescription medications often have a "life expectancy" of five years or more, that time period is really designated for the convenience of the pharmacist who purchases supplies from a wholesaler. It means that the contents of the sealed container will last for five years from the date of manufacture. Of course, the expiration date appears only on the large-sized containers purchased by pharmacies; the druggist does not usually include the manufacturer's expiration date on individual prescription labels, so you have no idea how long he or she has had the supply on hand before filling your prescription. Once the pharmacist has opened the container and begun using the contents to fill prescriptions, deterioration begins. Most pharmacists are careful to dispose of little-used drugs periodically in order not to sell ineffective or potentially harmful medicines. You may want to consider patronizing a high-volume pharmacy that has a fairly rapid turnover of its stock.

A good rule of thumb to follow is to discard and replace liquid medications that become cloudy or change color or any medication, liquid or tablets, whose odor changes markedly. Regardless of appearance, liquid medications should be discarded in about a month. The stability of some drugs—nitroglycerin is a good example—is fragile and may require special storage conditions or time limits. Purchasing large supplies of medications at one time, that is, more than you can reasonably expect to use quickly, can be a false economy if you end up throwing away an outdated portion. Discuss with your pharmacist just how long you may safely keep any medications, prescription or OTC, on hand. It may be wiser for you to purchase smaller quantities at more frequent intervals than to buy a "bargain" that you cannot use.

Your physician will usually prescribe a specific quantity of medicine when treating transitory illnesses such as bacterial infections. It is important that you take the full amount of medicine prescribed in order to ensure that the illness will not recur, even if the apparent symptoms abate rather quickly. The body can harbor infections for several days after outward signs of the illness disappear. Your doctor's prescription takes this into consideration and provides enough medicine to eliminate any lingering bacterial growth. You should never attempt to hold a little medicine back in case you (or worse, someone else in your fam-

Medication Storage Temperatures

Room temperature: generally 59–86°F (15–30°C)
Cool: generally 46–59°F (8–15°C)
Refrigerated: generally 36–46°F (2–8°C)
Cold: below 46°F (8°C)
Excessive heat: above 104°F (40°C)

Note: All medications should be protected from freezing or excessive heat, either of which could change the properties of the ingredients. Regardless of the specified storage temperature, you should always make sure all medicine containers are tightly sealed to prevent moisture from entering. Store all medicines away from light whenever possible.

ily) get sick again, for two reasons: the effectiveness of the medicine could change, or you could fail to rid your system of the bacteria causing your original problem.

Sometimes a physician might prescribe a pain-relieving medication that you may not use up because your discomfort is not so great that you need to use the drug. Do not keep the medicine around in case you have some other aches or pains sometime in the future. Drugs are prescribed for specific complaints at specific times for specific persons, and it is possible for your body to react differently to a drug taken at a later date. Any supply of medicine that you do not require should be safely disposed of once the reason for its prescription no longer exists.

Prescription drugs used to treat one person's ailments should never be used by anyone else. Some drug sensitivities can be detected only by tests, and taking another person's medicine could cause one to have a serious, even life-threatening, reaction.

SAVING MONEY

Naturally, as with any other purchase you make, you want the prescription drugs you buy to be as inexpensive as possible yet still safe and effective. Remember, however, that the key words are *safe* and *effective*. That has to be your most important consideration.

OTC Substitutes

Sometimes you can substitute a less expensive over-the-counter medicine for a prescription. Of course, this should be done only with the approval of your doctor. You should also discuss it with your pharmacist. For example, currently ibuprofen, a painkiller, is available both as a prescription drug and over the counter. The OTC brands were less expensive when they first entered the market. Then the manufacturers of the prescription versions lowered their prices to meet the competition. The OTC products contain only 200 mg of medication, however, while the prescription drugs come in dosages of 400 to 800 mg; you may have to take more of the OTC drug to achieve the desired effect. Thus, in this case the OTC may not be cheaper. It is always wise to check out the possibility of making substitutions with your pharmacist and your doctor.

Generic Drugs

Another way that you may be able to save money when buying prescription drugs is to investigate generic drugs. A generic drug is not protected by trademark registration. Thus a generic drug does not carry a brand name; often its name is simply the name of its ingredient(s) or a shortened version thereof.

A generic drug is often less expensive than a brand-name drug because it is not advertised as much. Ask your doctor to specify a generic drug on the prescription. Many states permit the pharmacist to fill a prescription with the least expensive equivalent, but in those areas where this is not allowed, the doctor can specify a generic substitute on the prescription.

It is important to remember that substituting a generic drug for a brand-name drug is not always possible or advisable. Some drugs are not available generically. Furthermore, some generic drugs are not noticeably less expensive than their trade-name counterparts. The most significant considerations, of course, are safety and effectiveness. Although the United States Food and Drug Administration (FDA), which regulates the pharmaceutical industry, claims that there is little or no evidence that there are differences between trade-name and generic drugs, some differences have surfaced between generics and certain brands. This may be of no consequence if the difference is small or irrelevant.

For example, if a generic does not begin working as quickly as its brand-name counterpart, this may not be important in a minor illness. If, however, the drug is being used to open air passages during an acute allergic reaction when time can mean life or death, you want the drug that acts most quickly. If you have questions, ask your doctor. Generic drugs may not be advisable for older persons.

In general, however, generic drugs are less expensive and as safe and effective as brand-name drugs. In fact, the reputation of generic drugs has improved in recent years, and as of 1984 there is legislation that will allow many more generic equivalents to be manufactured and marketed. Using generics is a good way to save money when you buy prescription drugs.

6

MANAGING SIDE EFFECTS

All medicines, whether they are sold by prescription only or over the counter as patent remedies, produce certain responses within the body. Ideally those responses will be beneficial and will have a therapeutic effect on a particular symptom or set of symptoms. That effect is called the drug's *indication*, or recommended use, as approved by the FDA. In other words, through testing and experimentation, research has found that a certain drug is indicated or suggested as an effective treatment for a certain condition.

Just as drugs offer desirable effects or benefits, however, they can also cause other responses that are unrelated to the illness being treated. These are called *side effects*.

Most side effects are a result of a drug's chemical activity and therefore are unavoidable. Many are undesirable, but most of them cause only minor inconvenience. Occasionally, however, a side effect becomes a serious condition or even a hazard in and of itself. These kinds of effects are often called *adverse reactions* to distinguish them from the more normal, expected, but unintended chemical activity of the drug while it works in the body. An adverse reaction is more serious than a side effect and may even become life-threatening. In fact, in some cases the risk from an adverse reaction to a drug far outweighs the benefit the drug offers.

How can you tell a relatively harmless side effect from a serious reaction?

STAYING INFORMED

Whenever you receive a prescription or an OTC recommendation from your doctor or health-care provider, you should be prepared to ask questions about the medication and its use. The questions should include these:

- Should I expect side effects from this medicine?
- If so, what is normal and predictable, and what warrants

medical attention?

• What is dangerous and needs emergency attention?

No matter how these questions are answered in your doctor's office, the time may come when you will wonder at home what you should do if you suddenly experience an unexpected response to a drug. You may wonder if the response is a side effect or if you are developing additional symptoms of the illness. You might consult your notes and instructions from your doctor but still be uncertain about whether the new symptoms you are having are a normal expected side effect or if you should be concerned enough to call the doctor.

To be on the safe side, you should always call your doctor if you are concerned or if you are not sure about how to interpret any new symptoms. Sometimes even a minor side effect can be minimized or eliminated by a change in dosage or by something as simple as taking the drug along with meals. If this is not possible, your doctor may be able to offer suggestions for managing the side effect. For example, some antibiotics can cause diarrhea as an expected side effect. This occurs because the antibiotic is designed to kill harmful bacteria, and in doing its job it also kills beneficial bacteria in the intestine. When the balance of bacteria in the intestine is disturbed, diarrhea can

occur. However, if you eat a carton of yogurt, the diarrhea will probably disappear because the fermented culture in the yogurt restores beneficial bacteria to the intestine.

If a side effect cannot be minimized or eliminated, your doctor may be able at least to give you some tips on how to cope with it. The accompanying chart will also offer some ideas on managing side effects.

OTC MEDICINES

It is imperative that you remember that over-the-counter medicines are just that—they are medicines and, like all medicines, are made up of certain chemicals. Of course, before appearing on the market, OTC remedies must be approved for general sale by the FDA and must contain certain information on their labels. If you have tried to read those labels, however, you have probably found that much of the information, particularly that which concerns the product's ingredients, is often printed in such small type and contains such forbidding chemical terms that it may be very difficult to read and understand.

Let's assume that you are taking a prescription medication for treatment of high blood pressure, and you develop a head cold. Would you know whether it

Coping with Drug Side Effects

Side Effect	What to Do
Blurred vision	Call your doctor.
Breathing difficulty	Call your doctor.
Constipation	Increase fluid intake; call your doctor if constipation lasts more than two days; do not take a laxative without asking doctor.
Diarrhea	Increase fluid intake; eat yogurt if you are taking an antibiotic; call your doctor if diarrhea lasts more than three days.
Dizziness	Avoid hazardous activities; lie down with your feet elevated; call your doctor if dizziness lasts more than two hours.
Drowsiness	Avoid activities requiring alertness; do not drive a car; call your doctor if your drowsiness persists.
Dry mouth	Eat candy, chew gum, or suck ice chips.
Dry nose, throat	Use a vaporizer; gargle salt water.
Fever	Call your doctor if fever is new symptom.
Headache	Call your doctor.
Itching; skin rash	Call your doctor.
Nasal congestion	Ask your doctor if it is all right to use nose drops.
Stomach upset	Ask your doctor if it is all right to take your medicine with food.

would be safe for you to purchase and use a decongestant that contains pseudoephedrine? (It probably would not.) Or perhaps you have found that aspirin taken for a headache often causes you to have an upset stomach. Would you recognize the acetylsalicylic acid listed among the ingredients of a patent remedy as being another name for aspirin? And would you know that some relatively simple oral antifungal medications, prescribed for the treatment of fungus infection of the skin or nails, can possibly cause liver damage in some patients, particularly women over 40 years of age?

WHEN TO CALL THE DOCTOR

Many side effects are self-limiting; that is, they disappear on their own accord without treatment. Others, however, require some management, and still others are warning signs that you should bring to the attention of your doctor. The following guidelines should help you decide which category a side effect falls into.

- Some drugs can cause dizziness, light-headedness, or a slight blurring of vision, all of which can be serious in an older person. Call your doctor. Meanwhile, try lying down with your feet higher than your head. You can sometimes overcome a moment of temporary dizziness by sitting down and placing your head between your knees. If you become light-headed, don't attempt to go up or down stairs, operate any kind of machinery, or do any cooking while the dizziness lasts. If dizziness becomes very pronounced or persists for more than two hours, call your doctor.

- Occasionally, a drug will cause a ringing, buzzing, or hollowness in the ears. This may be a symptom of aspirin overdose. Remember, many OTC remedies contain aspirin. If you are taking more than one kind of cold remedy at a time, you could possibly be receiving too much aspirin. These symptoms can also be caused by an ear infection.

- Always call your doctor at the first sign of breathing difficulty, noticeable vision difficulty, or any pain in your eyes. The antihistamines contained in most cold remedies and many OTC sleeping pills, for example, can increase the pressure within the eyes, a particularly dangerous reaction if you have any tendency toward glaucoma.

- Probably the most common side effects occur in the gastrointestinal system. This system consists of the mouth, esophagus, stomach, and small and large intestines. Many drugs can cause diarrhea, constipation, stomach upset, or dry mouth. Most of these side effects are self-limiting. As your body becomes accustomed to the drug, such effects will generally disappear. However, it is a good idea to call your doctor if any side effect in the gastrointestinal system persists for more than three days. Diarrhea can be managed by increasing your fluid intake to replace what is being lost. Do not use a diarrhea remedy or an antacid unless told by your doctor to do so. Some such medicines can actually increase the diarrhea. If diarrhea follows use of an antibiotic, you can try eating some yogurt to replace beneficial bacteria that the antibiotic has removed from the intestine. Constipation can also be handled by increasing the amount of fluids you normally drink. Extra water helps soften the stool and relieve constipation. If you have an upset stomach, check with your doctor to see whether taking your medicine along with milk might help prevent your pain or nausea. Sucking on ice chips will relieve a dry mouth.

- Drowsiness is also a common side effect. If you feel yourself becoming unusually drowsy soon after taking your medicine, avoid driving or operating any machinery; your normal awareness of hazards could be impaired.
- A headache should be reported to your doctor. It usually is not a serious side effect, but it is better to be on the safe side.
- If the drug you are taking causes you to have a stuffy nose, ask your doctor if you can use nose drops or a nasal spray. If your throat is dry, try a simple salt gargle (½ teaspoon salt to eight ounces of water). If you develop a sore throat or a fever a few days after starting a drug, call your doctor. This could be a sign that the drug has affected the body's immune system and an infection has set in.
- Some drugs can lead to photosensitivity, that is, unusual sensitivity to the sun. They include certain antibiotics, diuretics, tranquilizers, and oral diabetes medications. Although these drugs alone will not cause reactions, taking them and then being exposed to strong or prolonged sunlight can. This does not necessarily mean that you must avoid the sun altogether, but you should use a strong sunscreen, that is, one containing para-aminobenzoic acid (PABA), whenever you are going to be outside for a long period of time. Be sure, however, to check if PABA interacts with any other drugs you may be taking.
- Skin reactions such as itching, swelling, or a rash may indicate an allergy to a drug. If you develop any of these symptoms, call your doctor immediately. You may have to change drugs.

HIDDEN SIDE EFFECTS

Some side effects have no outward and apparent symptoms, but instead affect the body without your being aware of it. When this is known about a drug you are taking, your doctor may want to monitor your progress with laboratory tests, the only way of determining for certain whether you are experiencing the possible side effects. It is especially likely that your doctor may want to conduct periodic testing if you

Anaphylactic Shock

Anaphylactic shock is an extremely dangerous, life-threatening allergic reaction to a medication. It can also occur following insect sting. It is absolutely essential that immediate medical treatment for it be obtained.

Onset of symptoms of anaphylactic shock are apparent almost immediately after the offending medication is given or the insect sting occurs. If the reaction follows the injection of a medication, it will probably be a drug that a physician has just given, so it is likely that medical treatment will still be readily available. However, there is the possibility that you could already have left the doctor's office before the first symptoms become apparent or before you take the first dose by mouth.

Symptoms: General uneasiness and flushed face, followed by any or all of these rapidly developing conditions: skin welts (hives), itching skin, rapid heartbeat, breathing difficulty, sneezing, coughing, throbbing in the ears, vomiting, bowel and urine incontinence, convulsions. Shock, characterized by cold, clammy skin, weak and rapid pulse, and faintness, follows within a few minutes.

Treatment: Call an ambulance or emergency life squad immediately. Professional treatment is essential.

are taking certain medicines over a prolonged period of time.

A FINAL WORD

Any medicine, whether it is a pill, a capsule, or liquid that is swallowed or a lotion or cream applied externally, produces some kind of reaction within the body. Two drugs used simultaneously—even common, comparatively weak ones—can interact with each other to increase, decrease, or create a totally new effect on the body. Mixing or combining medicines without your physician's—or at least your pharmacist's—knowledge and advice can be a dangerous game, one that can have a significant effect on your health.

7

UNDERSTANDING DRUG INTERACTIONS

Anyone over the age of 50 years who takes one or more drugs and also eats and drinks should become familiar with food/drug and drug/drug interactions. Studies have shown that older people are more susceptible to drug reactions and interactions and are also more likely to be affected by them more seriously than are younger persons. Thus, it is important that you understand about interactions and how to prevent their occurrence.

FOOD/DRUG INTERACTIONS

Can you take your tetracycline antibiotic with a glass of milk? If you are taking a monoamine oxidase (MAO) inhibitor for high blood pressure or depression, do you have to avoid aged cheese or wine? The answers, respectively, are no and yes. First, the calcium in milk and other dairy products decreases the absorption of tetracycline. And second, MAO inhibitors may react with a sub-

stance called *tyramine* in cheese and wine, increasing blood pressure to dangerously high levels. These are only two food/drug interactions that are common. There is a difference between them, however. One, milk and tetracycline, causes the drug to be ineffective—in essence, useless. The other, MAO inhibitors and tyramine-containing foods, can be extremely dangerous. This example is vivid proof that you must be aware of possible food interactions with any medications you take.

The foods you eat can interact with your medications in several ways. Depending on the dosage and the individual's age and size, food can affect the way a drug is absorbed, either slowing down or speeding up the time the medicine takes to travel through the digestive system to the part of the body where it is needed. Or, as in the case of tetracycline and milk, a food can virtually prevent a drug from being absorbed properly. Often, too, taking some drugs with a carbonated beverage or an acidic fruit or vegetable juice may change those drugs' absorption rates by causing them to dissolve more quickly in the stomach rather than in the intestine where they are more readily absorbed into the bloodstream.

Food/drug interactions can also occur because of natural or added chemicals in the food that can render the drugs useless or, as is the case with the MAO inhibitors, outright dangerous. For example, licorice contains a substance that raises blood pressure. If you have high blood pressure, eating licorice may not only raise your blood pressure but may also counteract the effects of your high blood pressure medication. Brussels sprouts, cabbage, kale, rutabagas, soybeans, and turnips contain substances that work against thyroid hormone; therefore, if you are taking a thyroid hormone supplement, you should avoid large amounts of these foods.

DRUG/FOOD INTERACTIONS

So far we have been discussing how foods can interfere with the absorption or effectiveness of drugs. Drugs, however, can also interfere with the absorption and use of foods. Drugs can speed up the progress of nutrients through the intestinal system so that their value is lost to the body. Drugs can hinder absorption of nutrients or interfere with the body's ability to convert nutrients into usable forms. For example, a vitamin C or folic acid deficiency may occur in individuals who are using anticonvulsants to manage epilepsy, because these drugs increase the turnover rate of these vitamins in the body. The effects of some drugs on the wall of the intestine may inhibit absorption of nutrients; colchicine, a gout drug, and mineral oil, used in

Foods Containing Tyramine

aged cheese	chicken livers	sour cream
avocados	fermented foods	soy sauce
bananas	other wines in	yeast preparations,
beef liver	large amounts	including brewer's
beer	pepperoni	yeast
broad beans (fava)	pickled herring	yogurt
canned figs	salami	
Chianti wine	sherry	

MAO inhibitors are also suspected of reacting with cola drinks, chocolate, coffee, and raisins.

some nonprescription laxatives, both have this effect.

Other drugs may impair the body's production of special chemicals to convert nutrients into usable forms or may combine with the nutrient so that it is passed out of the body without being absorbed. This is a chemical process that occurs with the high blood pressure drug hydralazine and the tuberculosis drug INH, which prevent the body from using vitamin B_6. More commonly known, diuretics can deplete the body of potassium stores by pulling potassium out of the body along with water and salt.

DRUG/DRUG INTERACTIONS

If you are taking more than one medication, or if you are using a prescription along with a nonprescription preparation, you must take the time to find out the possible drug interactions among your medications. As a rule, older persons generally experience more drug reactions and interactions. Part of the reason for this is that more than eight out of 10 persons over 60 years of age have chronic health problems for which they are receiving medical care. In many cases more than one drug is needed, and the possibility of drug interaction is much greater when more than one drug is being taken.

The drugs most often associated with interactions include antibiotics, heart medicines, central nervous system drugs, diuretics, and diabetes medications. There are two primary ways drugs interact with each other: (1) one drug may increase or decrease the effects of the other, and (2) one drug may interfere with the absorption and use of the other drug. Both of these processes may be exaggerated by the aging process as well.

Can drug interaction be prevented? A comprehensive discussion with your doctor is necessary for you to answer this question. You must first tell your doctor about all of the drugs you are taking. You may think that, because your doctor prescribed the drugs, he or she should know exactly what you are taking. In some cases that may be true, but does your doctor know that you take an over-the-counter antacid every night before bed? What other nonprescription products do you use, either on a regular basis or only occasionally? Has another doctor been treating you—a specialist to whom your regular doctor referred you? Has this specialist prescribed a drug for you? Has your dentist given you any medicine? Has your foot doctor recommended a medication? All of these contingencies can lead to or contribute to a drug interaction. You should tell not only your regular doctor exactly what medications you use, but also your specialist, dentist, and foot doctor, and you should specify both over-the-counter medications and prescriptions from any of your other medical caregivers. As you can see, you and the information you share are the keys to preventing drug interactions.

You can also ask your doctor questions about your medicines:

- Will the interaction be eliminated if we change the dosage amount or time?
- Are there other dosage forms— sustained-release capsules, the transdermal patches, and so forth—that might alter the way the drug enters the body and therefore prevent or cause an interaction?
- Can one drug be discontinued without harmful consequences?
- Are any nonprescription items allowed? (Even something as common as aspirin can cause bleeding problems if used with anticoagulants, for example.)
- How can a drug/person interaction (discussed below) be prevented?

DRUG/PERSON INTERACTIONS

A drug/person interaction occurs when a person takes a medication incorrectly because of misunderstanding the directions, forgetfulness, or failure to comply. These interactions take place even though different drugs being taken by the person have been selected carefully to avoid interactions. These interactions may be preventable.

Below is a list of steps you can take to prevent this type of reaction. Again, as with any kind of interaction, you are the key to its prevention.

- Tell your doctor exactly what other drugs, prescription or nonprescription, you are taking. Take all your medications with you to the doctor's office.
- Ask for explicit details about how to use the medication. (See Chapter 5 for recommendations as to what to ask your doctor when you receive a prescription.)
- Discuss with your doctor or pharmacist methods of taking your medicine that will prevent mix-ups, missed doses, overdoses, or confusion. If you take several medications, you can purchase pillboxes with multi-

Drinking, Smoking, and Drugs

A good rule of thumb is to avoid alcohol whenever you are taking a prescription or nonprescription drug, unless you obtain your doctor's approval. Many drugs interact with alcohol, often in very dangerous ways. Others increase the effects of alcohol, which can also be potentially harmful, especially if you try to drive or operate possibly dangerous equipment. Remember, alcohol is a drug.

Nicotine in tobacco also is a drug and can interact with some other drugs. Often the effect of a medication is reduced in a smoker because the drug is eliminated more quickly than in nonsmokers. For example, smoking increases the liver's metabolism of some drugs, including theophylline, thus speeding the drug through the body. If you smoke, ask your doctor if smoking will interfere with any drugs you are taking.

Some drugs that do not mix well with alcohol:

- antibiotics
- anticoagulants
- antidepressants
- antihistamines
- diabetes drugs, including insulin
- high blood pressure medications
- monoamine oxidase inhibitors
- sedatives
- tranquilizers

Some drugs that do not mix well with smoking:

- antidepressants
- benzodiazepines
- bronchodilators
- insulin
- painkillers
- propranolol (beta blocker)
- tranquilizers

ple compartments that you can use to keep track of what you have or have not taken. Most people place a day's worth of medications in these boxes in the morning. Some can be marked with the time to take the particular medicine, and there are even pillboxes that buzz or ring at the appropriate time. If you are taking a medication on a short-term basis and are likely to forget a dose, set a timer or an alarm clock to remind you. Ask the doctor if your medications can be prescribed in such a way that most of them are physically distinct from the others in size, shape, and color. Sometimes an equivalent product can be substituted if it differs physically from some of your other medications.

- If you have trouble reading your prescription label, ask the pharmacist if he or she can provide you with larger type on the label.
- Use self-adhesive colored stickers on your medicine containers as a quick identification reference, particularly if you have trouble reading the label.
- Draw a clock with dosage times on the self-adhesive stickers for easy reference.
- Be certain to ask your doctor what to do if you miss a dose of any of your medicines.

If you adhere to these guidelines, you should be able to avoid drug/person interactions. A final suggestion: see Chapter 2 for suggestions on contacting your poison control center if you think you may have mistakenly taken too much of one or another of your medications.

8

PREVENTIVE MEDICINE

We are all familiar with immunizations and vaccinations for children against such ailments as measles, mumps, rubella, whooping cough, tetanus, diphtheria, and, of course, poliomyelitis. And from infancy children are given vitamins and dietary supplements to assure their proper and healthy development. But what about adults? Do such prevention needs disappear as we grow older? The answer is no: disease prevention and good health practices change among adults, but there is always the need to observe certain precautions.

In general, adults should be vaccinated against tetanus and diphtheria. Tetanus is a disease that is caused by bacteria entering the bloodstream through a cut or puncture wound in the skin. It causes constrictions of the muscles in the jaw, throat, and neck (sometimes called *lockjaw*) and can lead to impaired breathing or even asphyxiation. Diphtheria is also a bacteria-caused disease and is highly contagious. It produces a toxin that kills all the cells near the infection site, forming a membrane made of dead tissue cells on which the bacteria continue to grow. This very toxic substance enters the circulation, causing all body cells to weaken and finally to cease functioning. The heart and the kidneys are especially affected. Diphtheria symptoms and complications can progress rapidly and can be fatal.

Both tetanus and diphtheria are treatable, but, more importantly, both are preventable. Effective and safe vaccines that can eliminate the possibility of contracting either one are readily available. Unfortunately, despite these facts, only approximately 40 percent of adult Americans have been vaccinated against tetanus, and about 30 percent carry antibodies against diphtheria.

Age, of course, along with environmental conditions, occupations, general physical health, and other factors such as domestic or foreign travel all play roles in determining whether a person should be immunized against certain diseases. Older persons, for instance, should also be inoculated against influenza and pneumococcal infections, that is, diseases such as pneumonia that are caused by certain bacteria. Travel to foreign countries, or even to other areas of the United States, where health and environmental conditions are different from those at home, may necessitate additional disease-specific immunizations. Even temporary or permanent admission to an extended-care facility such as a nursing home may make vaccination against hepatitis B virus infection (HBV) advisable. Adult immunizations are much more specialized than children's and are more likely to produce reactions with other medications also being taken, so it is advisable to seek the advice of a professional health-care provider when planning protection against either common diseases or uncommon conditions.

INFLUENZA

Some illnesses that may be merely bothersome to children and younger adults can actually become dangerous to older persons, particularly those over 65. Influenza, for instance, may cause considerable discomfort to younger adults, but among older persons, including those in relatively good health, it can progress to pneumonia and other respiratory distress, even to the point of becoming life-threatening.

There are several different strains of influenza virus, and medications designed to protect against one variety may not be effective against another. Every year seems to bring a new virus or configuration of viruses for which it is necessary to devise new vaccines and immunization procedures. Check with your doctor about the advisability of receiving flu shots, particularly if you are over age 65 or if you are especially susceptible to such lingering complications as bronchitis, asthma, or pulmonary (lung) infections. Persons under treatment for cardiac conditions may be at risk in receiving influenza vaccinations.

Flu shots are generally given early in the fall and are often administered in two equal doses over a two-month period. They become effective against the disease within about two weeks and can sometimes cause relatively mild flulike reactions. Such reactions may be reduced somewhat by administering smaller amounts of the vaccine over a period of several days. Be certain to tell your physician if you have experienced discomfort or flu symptoms following previous vaccinations. Also, mention whether you have ever had any allergy to eggs or egg products, because the vaccine can cause a serious reaction where such sensitivity is present.

Annual booster shots for flu are advisable, but remember that influenza viruses mutate. Therefore, although your body develops an immunity to one strain of influenza that you have had or one for which you have received immunization, it is still possible for you to contract a totally new variety of the disease. Evidence does indicate, however, that flu shots can be effective—one study showed a nearly 80 percent mortality reduction among one group of elderly and chronically ill subjects who were inoculated against influenza over another unvaccinated group. Despite the widespread availability of influenza vaccines, the number of American adults who are at greatest risk if they contract flu but who have not been inoculated has been declining in recent years to the point that only about one-third are protected. Talk to your doctor and ask specific questions about a proper immunization program.

PNEUMONIA

Pneumococcal pneumonia is still one of the most common causes of death by infection in older people. Yet a very safe and effective vaccine is available.

This vaccine is manufactured by a new concept in vaccine formation. Since the body builds up defenses against the membrane of a bacterium, the vaccine is made from only the membrane of the pneumococcus bacterium. All or most of the protein of the bacteria is eliminated from the vaccine, which practically eliminates undesirable side effects from the vaccine.

The resulting vaccine offers so much protection that a second inoculation may never be needed. In fact, the body defenses are so increased by the one shot that the body will react quickly with a very red and sore arm if a second shot is given. Therefore, you should keep a record if you have had a pneumonia vaccination; make a note on your Medicare card or driver's license so that you will not receive a second vaccination.

This vaccine, of course, will not prevent viral, fungal or aspiration types of pneumonia.

AVOIDANCE OF IMMUNIZATIONS

If immunizations are available and safe, why do people, especially those most in need—the elderly and the chronically ill—avoid them? There are several reasons, ranging from a person's basic reluctance to get a shot to economic hardship to ignorance (yes, even on the part of a few physicians) about their effectiveness.

It is true that there have been occasional adverse reactions from vaccinations of all kinds, and some deaths have been reported as having been caused by certain vaccines. But vaccines and the techniques for their administration have been improved so much in recent years that the likelihood of a serious reaction occurring has been reduced to the point that it becomes almost statistically insignificant when weighed against the benefits enjoyed by the overwhelming majority of those who receive vaccinations. Also, because disease epidemics have decreased over the years, public consciousness has lessened regarding prevention of such dreaded illnesses as polio and diphtheria. That kind of complacency—the feeling that the threat no longer exists and that it is not necessary to protect oneself from "outdated" diseases—can, of course, lead to a recurrence of what was thought to be a disease of the past.

The reluctance by some insurance companies and by the federal government, under the provisions of Medicare, to pay for inoculations has also led to fewer people seeking immunizations and has resulted in a curious situation in which treatment of disease is compensated but prevention of the same disease is not. It is more expedient for many people, particularly those on fixed incomes, to take the chance that they will remain healthy rather than pay to receive inoculations.

Talk to your physician about the safety and effectiveness of immunizations. Ask for an explanation of how vaccinations work and how they affect your particular situation. Are you at higher risk now of contracting certain diseases than you were several years ago? Considering your general state of health, what kinds of precautions should you be taking to avoid illnesses?

NUTRITIONAL NEEDS

As people grow older, their nutritional needs change. They may be expending considerably less energy than they did when they were younger because of a slower, somewhat more sedentary lifestyle. Also, aging causes changes in metabolism, the process by which the body utilizes food, converting it from matter to energy. On top of everything else, a person's enjoyment of food may diminish as he or she grows older and the sense of taste begins to wane, and, if he or she lives alone, the rewards of preparing a well-balanced meal may not be seen as worth the effort required to do so. Snacking may become the primary means of eating.

Malnutrition among older persons is not at all uncommon, but it may not be immediately apparent to their friends or relatives. Malnutrition is not necessarily synonymous with starvation; rather, it is the lack of essential foods and the important substances they contain. And it does not always show up as the weight loss or general wasting with which we are familiar from seeing pictures of refugees or starving Third World populations. A person suffering from malnutrition may continue to appear relatively normal and well nourished while suffering such symptoms as skin and mouth sores that do not heal quickly, poor muscle tone, decreased reflexes, vision and other sensory abnormalities, and general fatigue. Often for older persons who may be suffering from some degree of malnutrition, it is not so much how much they are eating but what they are eating—or, more specifically, not eating—that is causing their problem.

The same basic food groups needed for good health that we all learned about as children—fresh fruits and vegetables, dairy products, grains and cereals, and meat and poultry items—are still essential for continued good health as we grow older. But the percentage of our diets that each represents may change a bit. For instance, it is probably wise for older persons to cut back somewhat on the amount of red meats (beef, veal, pork) that they eat and substitute in their place fish and lean chicken or turkey. Fresh, raw fruits and steamed or lightly cooked vegetables should become a larger part of one's overall daily diet, and whole grain breads and cereals should replace rich pastries and baked goods made from bleached and refined flours.

Just as it is possible to observe some outward characteristics of normal aging, it is important to understand that internal aging is also taking place. A simple indication of this can be seen in the decreased elasticity of the skin. Pinch a bit of skin on the back of an older adult's hand, and you will find that a small ridge remains before gradually receding. Do the same to a child's hand, and the pinched skin will immediately smooth out again. The same loss of elasticity, or tone, that appears in the skin also occurs within other organs of the body where it cannot be seen. The intestines, for example, slowly begin losing their tone as the body ages. The effect is that food may digest more slowly, resulting in changes in the ways in which the body receives and processes food substances. Some foods, perhaps including favorites enjoyed for years with no ill effects, may eventually become more than the slower digestive system can handle and must be eliminated from one's diet.

Calcium

One of the major health problems facing older persons today is osteoporosis, literally a condition characterized by bones that have become soft and porous instead of hard and firm. The condition causes the bones, particularly the long bones of the legs and arms, to become brittle and easily broken, sometimes by no more than a bump or a twist. Osteoporosis occurs in both sexes but is far more common in women, generally beginning gradually with the onset of menopause. The extent of the condition within the older population is demonstrated by the fact that more than $1 billion is spent every year for the treatment of hip fractures, one of the most common injuries suffered by those with the disease. Its painful effect can also be seen in the loss of height among older persons and the stooped stature sometimes referred to as "dowa-

ger's hump." Both of these conditions result from a gradual softening and deterioration of the vertebrae.

Osteoporosis is caused by a lack of calcium within the bones. Calcium is extremely important to the body because, in addition to keeping bones strong, it helps regulate the heart's contractions, aids in blood clotting, and is essential to nerve and muscle activity. As a rule, calcium is stored in the bones for use as the body needs it. The mineral must be maintained at a fairly constant level within the bones to assure a steady supply as the body requires it. If poor nutritional habits lower the consumption of calcium, thereby altering the stored amount available to supply various necessary functions, osteoporosis may occur. Of course the need for the mineral continues regardless of the amount of the calcium being consumed, so the body continues to draw the mineral from the bony storehouses. The result is thinning and weakening of the bones.

Usually, good nutritional practices—that is, a diet that contains a compensating amount of calcium-bearing foods—is sufficient for sustaining the proper amount of the mineral within the storage areas of the bones. Milk and other dairy products such as yogurt, cheeses, and ice cream are good calcium sources as are such vegetables as chard, cauliflower, and some of the stronger-tasting vegetables such as kohlrabi, beets, rutabagas, beans, turnips, carrots, and cabbage. A word of caution about dairy products, though: select only those items that are manufactured from milk. There are now some cheeses, ice cream, and a few other "dairy" products that are made from soya instead of milk.

While foods high in calcium content are essential for maintaining a proper calcium balance in the body, it is not enough that they be eaten alone. In order to be utilized by the body, calcium must be carried in solution through the bloodstream. Much of the calcium taken into the body is not converted into solution and passes through the intestines without being absorbed and utilized. Calcium requires vitamin D to convert it to a usable form; therefore, it is also necessary to make foods rich in that food element a part of your diet.

For those persons who cannot tolerate milk or milk products, calcium tablets are available. They may be prescribed by a physician or purchased over the counter at a drugstore; discuss your personal need with the pharmacist and ask his or her advice about dosage.

In general, if you maintain a balanced diet, selecting foods from all the food groups, you can maintain a healthy nutritional status. If you feel you are not eating properly, ask your doctor about vitamin and mineral supplements.

9

TIPS FOR
CAREGIVERS

Most persons who find themselves in the role of caregiver have had no preliminary experience, much less specific training, in attending to an ill person. Often the responsibility comes suddenly as the result of a heart attack or some other acute illness. Sometimes the caregiver finds himself or herself called upon to look after a spouse, parent, friend, or relative who cannot manage independently. It may be for a temporary recuperative period, or it may be a permanent situation. Whatever the conditions, it is up to the caregiver to familarize herself or himself with all of the patient's needs, the physician's recommendations, and the treatment program.

Actually, anyone who is under a physician's supervision for maintaining his or her own good health is a caregiver. As noted earlier, health care is a team effort involving both the patient and all of his or her health-care providers. Whether you are the patient yourself or you are caring for someone else, the information in this chapter may help you better understand the medical situation so that you can function more efficiently.

FOLLOWING THE DOCTOR'S ORDERS

When dealing with someone's illness or condition, whether it is temporary or permanent, chronic or acute, it is essential that you follow the instructions of the attending physician completely and conscientiously. Presumably his or her examination, questions, and previous care have revealed the nature of the patient's disease, overall health, and specific needs. It is the doctor's business to become informed about each patient and to exercise his or her professional judgment in designing an individual program of treatment. This is not to say, of course, that you should not ask questions and offer comments. You should. Anytime you feel there may be a particular bit of

Symptoms of Dehydration

- Infrequent urination
- Decreased amounts of urine
- Drowsiness
- Sunken eyes
- Rapid or slow breathing
- Dry mouth
- Skin remaining rigid when pinched gently
- Confusion
- Constipation

information, no matter how trivial, that could have an effect on the doctor's decisions about how to prescribe, it is your responsibility to make that information known. It could have a profound impact on the course of treatment.

When a doctor specifies that a drug be taken according to a certain schedule, it is important to follow those directions. Doses of some medicines, if given too close together, can produce overdoses. If given in doses too far apart, some other medicines cannot perform the action for which they are intended. Occasionally prescriptions carry instructions to take the medicine until it is gone. When a drug carries that direction, there is a reason for it. Antibiotics, for example, may make the symptoms of infection disappear within a couple of days even though the cause of the infection still exists but only a portion of the medicine has been taken. Stopping the medication too soon may allow the infection to recur and make it necessary for the doctor to prescribe a stronger antibiotic.

Some people see no reason to take their prescribed medication if they don't feel sick. Again, stopping a medicine without first consulting the doctor can be a mistake. For those persons with high blood pressure, for instance, it is important to take an antihypertensive drug continuously even though such symptoms as headache and dizziness have disappeared temporarily. Hypertension is a disease that may give no outward indication of its seriousness, thus informing its victim that it is time to take a pill.

MEMORY HELPERS

If it is your responsibility to help someone adhere to a prescribed medication schedule, write down exactly what it is you are supposed to do. How often are you expected to give each medicine? Should you give it with food or between meals? What kinds of reactions should you watch for? Is it all right for the patient to smoke or drink alcoholic beverages while on a particular medication?

If you have several pills to give or to take during the day, ask your pharmacist to show you a compartmentalized medication reminder box. These handy containers are divided into separate spaces for each day of the week so that you can lay out an entire week's worth of tablets all at one time. Some containers have one-day compartments that are further divided to enable you to tell at a glance whether you have given (or taken) all the necessary pills during the course of a day.

It is best not to put different kinds of pills into a single bottle because of the possibility of overlooking one at medication time. What you might do each morning, though, is to put all those pills to be taken at the same time in a separate envelope or bottle and mark on it the medication time. Do this for as many administration times as are prescribed during the day.

For those who find it especially difficult to remember when to give or take medicines, there is a pill container on the market that contains an alarm clock. Once

Diet to Treat Diarrhea

- Commercial mineral and electrolyte solutions
- Flavored gelatin water
- Flavored gelatin
- Diluted beef bouillon
- Small amounts of lean beef or lamb
- Boiled chicken
- Soft- or hard-boiled egg
- Cooked rice
- Dry baked or boiled potato
- Fresh banana
- Fresh apple
- Toast or crackers and jelly

preset, it buzzes and flashes a light whenever medication times roll around again. Ask your pharmacist about ordering one if the store does not stock them.

For safety's sake, every medicine container should be labeled with the person's name for whom the contents have been prescribed. This includes bottles, compartmentalized containers, portable medicine chests, and purse or pocket pillboxes.

OTHER CAREGIVERS

There may be times when you will turn over your caregiver responsibilities to someone else. You should prepare for those times by writing out clear and precise instructions and taking time to go over them thoroughly with whomever you are leaving in charge. Don't expect "sitters" to figure out what should be done; tell them and write it down.

Include in your instructions any dietary restrictions; medication times, with exact directions for administering each medicine; a list of all medicines, prescription or OTC, the patient is using; all nondrug treatments; periodic routine test procedures such as blood pressure or urine checks; and any personal habits, preferences, or idiosyncrasies of the patient. Be sure to add specific descriptions of danger signs to be aware of. Look over your list once a month or so to see if it needs to be updated.

Don't forget to discuss emergency procedures with the sitter, even if you plan to be gone for only an hour or so. Show the sitter what to do in case of a fire and tell him or her whom to call if anything goes wrong. You should keep a list of important telephone numbers (emergency squad, doctor, drugstore, poison control

---

Diet to Treat Constipation

- All fruits (except bananas and apples), especially if eaten with skin on
- All vegetables, especially if eaten raw (except peeled potatoes)
- Whole grain cereals and breads
- Unrefined sugars—honey, molasses, brown sugar
- More water, expecially a 12-ounce glass of warm water upon arising in the morning

center, and family members and neighbors) posted next to every telephone in the home. Go over the list with the sitter before leaving home. Never leave an elderly patient in the care of a child who is unable to handle any emergency situation that may arise. For instance, do not entrust the care of a grandparent to a young child who could not move the patient in case of a fire or other emergency.

PART II: MEDICATION PROFILES

I n this section you will find descriptions, called *profiles*, of some commonly used medications. The profiles have been categorized as either prescription drugs (Chapter 10), for which your doctor must write a prescription, or over-the-counter products (Chapter 11), which you can buy without a prescription.

Each profile gives the most important information about a drug. By reading a drug's profile, you will learn what to expect from that drug, in terms of either its benefits or its adverse effects. Many persons prefer to read a drug's profile before filling a prescription so that they can clarify any points of confusion or ask knowledgeable questions of their pharmacist.

To use the profiles most efficiently, you should understand the significance of each category in the profile. Each prescription drug profile contains the following information:

• *Name of Drug.* Each drug is listed by either its brand name or its generic name, which is usually the name of its ingredient(s). A general rule of thumb to remember is that brand names begin with a capital letter and generic names with a lower-case letter.

• *Ingredients.* This section lists the principal chemical components of the medication.

• *Equivalent Product(s).* This category lists all drugs that are chemically the exact same formulation as the drug being profiled. Again, if a drug is available as a generic, the generic name will not be capitalized. If your doctor has prescribed a drug that is available generically, ask to have the prescription request the generic equivalent; it may be cheaper. Remember, however, that not all generic drugs are exactly equivalent to trade-name drugs; this is information you should ask your pharmacist about.

• *Used For.* This section describes what the drug is prescribed for.

• *Dosage Form and Strength.* The forms of the drug (tablets, liquids, capsules, and so forth) are listed, along with each form's strength or concentration of active ingredients. In a few cases, not all of the available forms of a drug are listed; in such cases, there are forms or strengths that are generally recommended only for use with children.

• *Storage.* This information enables you to store your drug properly for maximum effectiveness and safety.

• *Before Using This Drug, Tell Your Doctor.* This section tells you what your doctor needs to know about you before a medication is prescribed or used. Some medications are the preferred choice of treatment for a certain illness, but they should not be used for a person with a history of hypertension, as an example. The doctor must also know about any other drugs you are currently taking and about any allergies or family history of allergies. This information is extremely important.

• *This Drug Should Not Be Used If.* Here you will learn when a drug should not be used and under what circumstances a drug's use is inappropriate or even hazardous.

• *How to Use.* This section offers tips on taking the drug alone or as part of a compound. You will learn if you should take the drug on an empty stomach or with food. You will read about

dosage intervals. In short, this category will help you give or take the medicine in the most effective and safe way.

• *Time Required for Drug to Take Effect.* By knowing this information, you will be able to evaluate the effectiveness of the drug you are taking.

• *Missing a Dose.* This section instructs you in what to do if you forget to take your medicine. Even with these guidelines, this is a question to ask your doctor so that you are absolutely sure of what to do in such a situation.

• *Symptoms of Overdose.* If you take too much medication, the symptoms listed in this section will alert you to the danger of overdose. Many of these symptoms will also appear in the "Serious adverse reactions" section.

• *Side Effects.* This category is divided into two sections: minor and expected and serious adverse reactions. The minor side effects are those that are unavoidable and that also tend to disappear as you become accustomed to the drug or as your dosage is adjusted by your doctor. Do not expect that all of these effects will automatically occur, but if they do, you will know that they are not too serious. On the other hand, if minor side effects persist or seem unusually severe, call your doctor. There is no sense in tolerating a side effect, no matter how minor, that is more uncomfortable than the symptom the drug is supposed to be treating if it can be avoided. Sometimes a change in dosage will eliminate these side effects.

Those effects listed under "Serious adverse reactions" always warrant a call to your doctor. If you are taking a prescription drug and experience an adverse reaction, do not automatically stop taking the drug—sometimes stopping a drug suddenly is as dangerous as the adverse effects it is causing—but do call your doctor immediately. The doctor may have to weigh the benefit of the drug against the risk of its adverse effects. Again, too, perhaps changing the dosage will eliminate the problem.

- *Effects of Long-Term Use.* This information will help you be aware of the benefit-versus-risk question concerning the drug.
- *Habit-Forming Possibility.* This section informs you about the possibility of your developing a physical or psychological dependence on a drug.
- *Precautions and Suggestions.* This category is divided into three sections: foods and beverages, other medicines, and other miscellaneous informa-

tion you should know about the drug. The food and beverages section tells you about any restrictions in regard to these items. Even if you do not ordinarily drink alcoholic beverages, you should be aware that some over-the-counter medications contain alcohol. To be on the safe side, always assume that alcohol will interact with any drug. The other two subsections of this category explain drug interactions and other activities that may enhance or decrease the effects of a drug. You will also find tips about using the drug.

- *Medical Tests.* Here you will find out if a drug will interfere with the results of a test or if your doctor will want to perform medical tests on you during the drug therapy to monitor the progress. Don't forget to tell anyone recommending or performing a medical test that you are taking medication. Also, don't forget about dentists and other specialists and health-care providers.

The over-the-counter drug profiles include most of the same categories of information as above. Those categories referring to specific treatment by a physician ("Before Using This Medication . . ." and "Medical Tests") have been eliminated because they generally relate only to prescriptions or to physicians' recommendations. The "Time Required . . ." category does not appear in this section because OTC medications are generally purchased to treat short-term symptoms of nonacute ailments, not the causes of the ailments themselves, as is more often the case with prescription drugs. Again, it must be emphasized that even with OTC products you must be alert to your reactions. These profiles will help you, but always call your health-care provider if you question anything about an OTC drug and the effect it is having on you.

10

PRESCRIPTION DRUGS

ALDOMET

Ingredient(s): methyldopa

Equivalent Product(s): methyldopa (generic)

Used for: treatment of high blood pressure

Dosage Form and Strength: tablets—125 mg, 250 mg, 500 mg; oral suspension—250 mg per 5 ml

Storage: Store in a dry, tightly closed container.

Before Using This Drug, Tell Your Doctor: about any history of liver disease, kidney disease, anemia, diabetes, heart disease, stroke, Parkinson's disease, gout, mental depression, or pheochromocytoma. Tell your doctor if you are undergoing dialysis. Also tell your doctor about any drugs, prescription or nonprescription, you are taking and about any allergies you have or any family history of allergies.

This Drug Should Not Be Used If: you are allergic to it or have any liver disease, including hepatitis or cirrhosis.

How to Use: Take Aldomet with water at the same time or times each day as directed. Measure the liquid form with a medical teaspoon.

Time Required for Drug to Take Effect: It may take two to four weeks of monitoring and dose adjustment before this drug maintains blood pressure at the desired measurements.

Missing a Dose: Take the missed dose as soon as you remember, but if it is almost time for the next dose, do not take the missed dose at all. Instead, return to your regular schedule. Do not double the next dose.

Symptoms of Overdose: extreme drowsiness, weakness, exhaustion, dizziness, fainting, falling, light-headedness, stupor, confusion, slow and weak pulse

Side Effects:

Minor and expected:
- drowsiness, fatigue, weakness, headache (all of which may occur during the first few weeks and then disappear), nasal stuffiness, dry mouth, dizziness

Serious adverse reactions (CALL YOUR DOCTOR):
- light-headedness sitting or standing up, prolonged fatigue, muscle pain or spasms, joint pain, decreased sexual interest, impotence, breast enlargement in men and women, milk production, nausea, constipation, diarrhea, sore or dark tongue, rash, heartbeat irregularities, fever, sore throat, chills, unusual bleeding or bruising, swelling of feet or legs, sleeplessness, confusion, mental disturbances, nightmares, memory impairment, chest pain, unusual body movements, shakiness, severe stomach pain with severe vomiting or diarrhea, yellow discoloration of the skin and eyes, pale-colored stools, dark-colored urine.

Effects of Long-Term Use: hemolytic anemia (a deficiency of red blood cells and hemoglobin, which carry oxygen throughout the body), retention of water with subsequent weight gain, development of "on and off again" effect of drug's action

Habit-Forming Possibility: none

Precautions and Suggestions:

Foods and beverages:
- No food restrictions, although your doctor may advise you about salt and other minerals in your diet to manage your high blood pressure.
- Ask your doctor before drinking any alcoholic beverages while taking this drug.

Other medicines, prescription and nonprescription:
- Avoid cough, cold, allergy, sinus, or weight control preparations, both prescription and over-the-counter, except under medical supervision while taking Aldomet.
- Aldomet may interact with other high blood pressure medications, antidiabetic medications, lithium, and haloperidol.
- This drug may also interact with drugs for parkinsonism, oral anticoagulants, digoxin, beta blockers, antidepressants, ephedrine, and phenothiazines.
- The drug may interact with anesthetics; tell your doctor or dentist, before any surgery or use of anesthetic, that you are taking Aldomet.

Other:

- The drug can interfere with blood transfusions; if you are giving or receiving blood, tell the medical attendant that you are taking Aldomet.
- Do not discontinue this drug without consulting your doctor; high blood pressure can return quickly, possibly within 48 hours.
- If this drug makes you drowsy, do not engage in any activity that requires alertness, including driving a car or operating potentially dangerous machinery.
- Use caution when exercising; exercise may lower blood pressure and in combination with Aldomet may reduce pressure too much. On the other hand, isometric exercise in combination with Aldomet may increase blood pressure. Discuss exercise with your doctor.
- Hot weather, heat (as in the workplace), and fever accompanying illness can reduce blood pressure. You may have to have your doctor adjust the dosage if hot weather, heat, or fever affects you.
- If you are over 60 years old, your doctor will probably start you out with small doses and monitor your blood pressure frequently. Sudden and rapid lowering of blood pressure may lead to stroke or heart attack in this age group. Also, using Aldomet in this age group may produce parkinsonism or intensify existing parkinsonism. If you notice symptoms of parkinsonism (masklike face, shakiness, trembling in limbs, stiffness, rigid posture and gait), contact your doctor.
- The drug can have powerful effects on older people; be certain that you understand the use of this drug and cooperate with your doctor or health-care provider.
- The ability of older people to absorb the generic form of this drug has been variable. This may be corrected in the future because the problem lies with the material mixed with the drug to make the pill.

Medical Tests:

- This drug can interfere with laboratory tests, including those for gout and pheochromocytoma.
- If your doctor orders a Coombs test for anemia, tell him or her that you are taking Aldomet; this drug may cause a false positive result when no disorder is present.
- Your doctor may want to monitor your progress on this drug with regular blood and urine tests, especially for blood cell and liver function.
- Any drug may affect the results and accuracy of a medical test. If a doctor recommends a medical or laboratory test for any condition, inform the doctor that you are taking this drug.

ALDORIL

Ingredient(s): hydrochlorothiazide and methyldopa

Equivalent Product(s): none

Used for: treating high blood pressure

Dosage Form and Strength: tablets—15 mg hydrochlorothiazide, 250 mg methyldopa (Aldoril-15); 25 mg hydrochlorothiazide, 250 mg methyldopa (Aldoril-25); 30 mg hydrochlorothiazide, 500 mg methyldopa (Aldoril D30); 50 mg hydrochlorothiazide, 500 mg methyldopa (Aldoril D50)

Storage: Store in a dry, tightly closed container.

Before Using This Drug, Tell Your Doctor: if you have liver disease, diabetes, or a history of kidney disease, gout, lupus erythematosus, anemia, stroke, heart disease, asthma, Parkinson's disease, mental depression, bladder disorders or urination difficulties, pancreas disorders, or a tumor of the adrenal gland. Tell your doctor if you are undergoing dialysis. Also tell your doctor about any drugs, prescription or nonprescription, you are taking and about any allergies you have, especially to sulfa drugs, or a family history of allergies.

This Drug Should Not Be Used If: you are allergic to it or to sulfa drugs, if you have liver disease, including hepatitis and cirrhosis, or if you cannot urinate properly.

How to Use: Take with food or milk at the same time or times each day as directed.

Time Required for Drug to Take Effect: It may take two to four weeks of monitoring and dose adjustment before this drug can be determined to be maintaining blood pressure at desired measurements.

Missing a Dose: Take the missed dose as soon as you remember, but if it is almost time for the next dose, do not take the missed dose at all. Instead, return to your regular schedule. Do not double the next dose.

Symptoms of Overdose: extreme drowsiness, weakness, exhaustion, dizziness, fainting, falling, light-headedness, stupor, confusion, slow and weak or rapid pulse, muscle pain and cramping, nausea, vomiting, extreme dry mouth, thirst, lethargy

Side Effects:

Minor and expected:
- drowsiness, fatigue, weakness, headache (all of which may occur during the first few weeks and then disappear), light-headedness sitting or standing up, nasal stuffiness, dry mouth, dizziness, increased urination, loss of appetite, upset stomach, abdominal bloating, constipation, stomach cramping, increased sensitivity to sunlight

Serious adverse reactions (CALL YOUR DOCTOR):
- prolonged fatigue, muscle pain or spasms, joint pain, decreased sexual interest, impotence, breast enlargement in men and women, milk production, nausea, diarrhea, sore or dark tongue, rash, hives, itching, heartbeat irregularities, fever, sore throat, chills, unusual body movements, unusual bleeding or bruising, swelling of feet or legs, sleeplessness, tingling in fingers or toes, confusion, mental disturbances, nightmares, memory impairment, chest pain, weakness, restlessness, shakiness, severe stomach pain with severe nausea and vomiting or diarrhea, yellow discoloration of skin and eyes, pale-colored stools, dark-colored urine, difficulty breathing, blurred vision, runny nose, flushing, weight loss or gain

Effects of Long-Term Use: hemolytic anemia (a deficiency of red blood cells and hemoglobin, which carry oxygen throughout the body); imbalance of the water, salt, and potassium levels of blood and body tissue; development of "on and off again" effect of drug's action; possible development of diabetes in those susceptible to developing it

Habit-Forming Possibility: none

Precautions and Suggestions:

Foods and beverages:
- Your doctor may recommend a diet low in sodium and high in potassium while you are taking this drug. Ask your doctor to suggest foods to meet your diet requirements.
- Avoid large amounts of licorice while taking this drug.
- Ask your doctor if you can drink alcoholic beverages while using this drug.

Other medicines, prescription and nonprescription:
- Avoid cough, cold, allergy, sinus, painkiller, or weight control preparations, both prescription and nonprescription, except under medical supervision while taking Aldoril.

- Aldoril may interact with other high blood pressure medications, antidiabetic medicines, barbiturates, narcotics, calcium salts or vitamin D, sulfa drugs, quinidine, gout drugs (allopurinol, probenecid), indomethacin, cholestyramine, colestipol, lithium, and haloperidol.
- This drug may also interact with drugs for parkinsonism, oral anticoagulants, steroid drugs, norepinephrine, digoxin, beta blockers, antidepressants (especially monoamine oxidase inhibitors and tricyclic antidepressants), some diuretics, amphetamines, ephedrine, and phenothiazines.
- The drug may interact with anesthetics; tell your doctor or dentist before any surgery or any use of an anesthetic that you are taking Aldoril.
- Be certain to tell your doctor you are taking digitalis; careful monitoring is necessary if digitalis and Aldoril are taken at the same time.

Other:
- The drug can interfere with blood transfusions; if you are giving or receiving blood, tell the medical attendant that you are taking Aldoril.
- Do not discontinue this drug without consulting your doctor; high blood pressure can return quickly.
- If this drug makes you drowsy, do not engage in activities that require alertness, such as driving a car or operating potentially dangerous machinery.
- Use caution when exercising; exercise may lower blood pressure and in combination with Aldoril may reduce pressure too much. Also, avoid strenuous exercise or any activity (hot showers, saunas, etc.) that causes you to perspire heavily; this adds to the diuretic effect of this drug and lowers blood pressure too much. On the other hand, isometric exercise in combination with Aldoril may increase blood pressure. Discuss exercise with your doctor.
- If you develop a sensitivity to sunlight while using this drug, limit your exposure to sun and wear protective clothing and a sunscreen.
- If you develop an illness with severe diarrhea or vomiting that causes fluid loss, call your doctor.
- If you are over 60 years old, your doctor will probably start you out with small doses and monitor your blood pressure frequently. Sudden and rapid lowering of blood pressure in this age group may lead to stroke or heart attack. Also, using Aldoril in this age group may produce parkinsonism or intensify existing parkinsonism. If you notice symptoms of parkinsonism (masklike face, shakiness,

trembling in limbs, stiffness, rigid posture and gait), contact your doctor.
- Hot weather, heat (as in the workplace), and fever accompanying illness can reduce blood pressure. You may have to have your doctor adjust the dosage if hot weather, heat, and fever affect you.
- The drug can have powerful effects in older people; be certain that you understand the use of this drug and that you cooperate with your doctor or health-care provider.

Medical Tests:

- The drug can interfere with laboratory tests, including those for gout, pheochromocytoma, thyroid and parathyroid function, blood ammonia levels, and urinary steroid and catecholamine determinations. If your doctor suggests any of these tests, tell him or her that you are taking Aldoril.
- If your doctor orders a Coombs test, remind him or her that you are taking Aldoril; this drug may cause a false positive result when no disorder is present.
- Your doctor may want to monitor your progress on this drug with regular blood and urine tests, especially for blood cell counts, liver or kidney function, uric acid (a factor in gout), and blood sugar.
- Any drug may affect the results and accuracy of a medical test. If a doctor recommends a medical or laboratory test for any condition, inform the doctor that you are taking this drug.

AMOXICILLIN (GENERIC)

Ingredient(s): amoxicillin

Equivalent Product(s): Amoxil, Larotid, Polymox, Sumox, Trimox, Utimox, Wymox

Used for: treatment of bacterial infections, including infections of the ear, nose, throat, lower respiratory tract, skin, and genitourinary tract

Dosage Form and Strength: capsules—250 mg, 500 mg; chewable tablets—125 mg, 250 mg; oral suspension—50 mg per 1 ml, 125 mg per 5 ml teaspoon, 250 mg per 5 ml teaspoon; drops—50 mg per ml

Storage: Keep liquid forms in the refrigerator. Store all forms in tightly closed containers.

Before Using This Drug, Tell Your Doctor: about any asthmatic or allergic reaction you have had to penicillin or any other antibiotics.

Also, tell your doctor if you are allergic by nature or have ever had hay fever, hives, skin rashes, or any other allergic reactions to anything. Inform your doctor if you have ever been diagnosed as having liver or kidney problems. Be sure to tell your doctor about any other medicines (prescription or nonprescription) that you are taking.

This Drug Should Not Be Used If: you have had an allergic reaction to any form of penicillin or have had a previous reaction to amoxicillin.

How to Use: Take as directed by your doctor, usually at evenly spaced intervals around the clock. The drug can be taken with or without food. If you are using the oral suspension, shake the bottle well before measuring and measure the dose with a marked or medical teaspoon—an ordinary kitchen teaspoon is not an accurate measure. If you are giving the drops to a very elderly or confused person, measure the medicine in a marked dropper and release the solution directly into the inside of the person's cheek. The drops can also be mixed with milk, fruit juice, water, or ginger ale and taken immediately. If you do this, you must be certain that the person swallows the entire drink to receive the full dose of medicine.

Time Required for Drug to Take Effect: usually two to five days, depending upon the type and severity of infection being treated. However, you should continue taking the medication for the full time prescribed by your doctor even if you seem well; otherwise, the infection may return.

Missing a Dose: Take the missed dose immediately, but if it is almost time for the next dose, wait to give the next dose until about halfway through the regular interval betwen doses. For example, if you are to take a dose at 8:00 A.M., 4:00 P.M., and midnight, and remember at 3:00 P.M. that you forgot the 8:00 A.M. dose, take the missed dose at 3:00 P.M. but wait until about 8:00 P.M. to take the 4:00 P.M. dose. Then return to your regular schedule at midnight. Do not skip a dose or double the dose.

Symptoms of Overdose: possible severe and persistent nausea, vomiting, and/or diarrhea

Side Effects:

Minor and expected:
- diarrhea, nausea

Serious adverse reactions (CALL YOUR DOCTOR):
- hives, itching (especially in genital or anal area), or skin rash; difficult breathing; fever; joint pain; sore throat; dark-colored

tongue; yellow-green stools; sores in the mouth; severe and persistent nausea, vomiting, or diarrhea

Effects of Long-Term Use: possibility of superinfection—that is, a second infection in addition to the infection being treated. A superinfection is caused by bacteria and other organisms that are not susceptible to or affected by the drug being used to treat the original infection. Thus, these organisms, usually held in check by the beneficial bacteria destroyed by the drug, grow unchecked and cause a second infection that may require treatment with a different drug.

Habit-Forming Possibility: none

Precautions and Suggestions:

Foods and beverages:
• No restrictions.

Other medicines, prescription and nonprescription:
• Antacids and other antibiotics reduce the absorption and effect of amoxicillin.
• Amoxicillin also interacts with the gout drug probenecid.

Other:
• If mild diarrhea is a side effect, ask your doctor if you can eat yogurt. The beneficial bacteria in yogurt replace the intestine's natural beneficial bacteria that have been reduced or eliminated by amoxicillin.
• This drug should be taken for the full length of time recommended by your doctor even if you seem to have recovered. Otherwise, the infection may return and be more difficult to treat the second time.
• Do not use the medication beyond the expiration date on the label. As a general rule of thumb, discard after 14 days any unused liquid medication that has been refrigerated.
• If you ever have any doubts about how you are reacting to a medicine, call your doctor.

Medical Tests:

• Your doctor may recommend blood counts or liver or kidney function tests during treatment with this drug in order to monitor your progress.
• If amoxicillin is being used to treat a sexually transmitted disease, your doctor may want to perform diagnostic tests for from several months to two to three years.
• Any drug may affect the results and accuracy of a medical test. If a doctor recommends a medical or laboratory test for any condi-

tion, inform the doctor that you are taking amoxicillin before the test is performed.

ATIVAN

Ingredient(s): lorazepam

Equivalent Product(s): none

Used for: relief of anxiety, anxiety associated with depression, tension, and sleeplessness

Dosage Form and Strength: tablets—0.5 mg, 1 mg, 2 mg

Storage: Store in a dry, light-resistant, tightly closed container.

Before Using This Drug, Tell Your Doctor: if you have heart, liver, or kidney disease; epilepsy; a history of alcoholism or drug abuse; myasthenia gravis; glaucoma; parkinsonism; lung problems; stomach problems; or severe mental illness. Tell your doctor if you are emotionally depressed. Also tell your doctor about any drugs, prescription or nonprescription, you are taking and about any allergies you have or any family history of allergies.

This Drug Should Not Be Used If: you are allergic to its ingredient or to any other similar drug (in the drug family called *benzodiazepine*), if you have narrow-angle glaucoma, or if you have a severe mental illness.

How to Use: Take this drug with food or a full glass of water.

Time Required for Drug to Take Effect: The action of the drug usually begins within 30 minutes and peaks two to six hours later, depending on the dose. It may take two or three days before the drug's full effect is reached.

Missing a Dose: If you remember within an hour of the missed dose's normal time, take the missed dose. If more than an hour has passed, wait until the next scheduled dosage time. Do not double the dose.

Symptoms of Overdose: extreme drowsiness, confusion, lethargy, loss of muscle coordination, stupor, deep sleep, coma

Side Effects:

Minor and expected:
- drowsiness, lethargy, nausea, constipation, diarrhea, vomiting,

heartburn, dry mouth, loss of appetite, increased salivation, weight gain, headache, menstrual irregularities

Serious adverse reactions (CALL YOUR DOCTOR):
- confusion, extreme drowsiness or weakness, light-headedness, difficult urination, breathing problems, sore throat and fever, unsually rapid or slow heartbeat, decreased hearing, sleeping problems, vivid dreams, depression, hallucinations, irritability, sores in mouth, rash, itching, hives, unusual excitement or nervousness, stomach pain, yellow discoloration of skin and eyes, unsteadiness, slurred speech, unusual fatigue, blurred vision, restlessness, tremor, difficulty in concentrating, dizziness, muscle spasms, difficulty in swallowing, bladder control problems, loss of interest in sex, nasal congestion, breast enlargement in men, joint pain

Effects of Long-Term Use: physical and/or psychological dependence, impairment of blood cell production, impaired liver function. This drug is intended for short-term use only; your doctor may not want you to take it for more than six weeks without evaluating your condition and assessing the continued need for the drug.

Habit-Forming Possibility: This drug can cause physical and/or psychological dependence if continued for a long period of time.

Precautions and Suggestions:

Foods and beverages:
- No restrictions on foods.
- Avoid alcohol while taking Ativan.
- Avoid large amounts of drinks containing caffeine; caffeine will diminish the sedative effects of Ativan. Caffeine is found in coffee, tea, colas, and chocolate.

Other medicines, prescription and nonprescription:
- Ativan may interact with central nervous system depressants, including sedatives, narcotics, barbiturates, tranquilizers, pain relievers, sleeping drugs, antihistamines, allergy and asthma medications, and antidepressants (including monoamine oxidase inhibitors).
- Ativan may also interact with anticonvulsants, levodopa, anticoagulants, and lithium.
- Do not use over-the-counter preparations for colds, allergy, cough, sinus, sleep, or weight reduction; all can possibly increase the sedative effect of Ativan.
- Smoking tobacco can affect the action of the drug in the body.

Other:

- *Do not* stop taking this drug abruptly; stopping Ativan without tapering off under medical supervision may lead to a withdrawal period.
- Do not exercise strenuously until you have determined how the drug affects your body. For example, if the drug causes you to urinate a greater than usual amount, you want to avoid exercise that causes excessive sweating so that you maintain normal water levels in the body.
- If this drug makes you drowsy or dizzy, avoid tasks that require alertness, such as driving a car or operating potentially dangerous machinery.
- The drug can have powerful effects in older people; be certain that you understand the use of this drug and that you cooperate with your doctor or other health-care provider.

Medical Tests:

- You doctor may want to perform periodic blood tests and liver and kidney function tests to monitor your progress while taking this drug.
- Ativan can affect the results of some laboratory tests.
- Any drug may affect the results and accuracy of a medical test. If a doctor recommends a medical or laboratory test for any condition, inform the doctor that you are taking this drug.

AUGMENTIN

Ingredient(s): amoxicillin and potassium clavulanate

Equivalent Product(s): none

Used for: infections of the ear, throat, sinuses, skin and skin structure, lower respiratory tract, and urinary tract caused by bacteria that have become resistant to penicillin and other antibiotics

Dosage Form and Strength: tablets—250 mg amoxicillin, 125 mg potassium clavulanate; 500 mg amoxicillin, 125 mg potassium clavulanate; pediatric oral suspension—125 mg amoxicillin, 31.25 mg potassium clavulanate; 250 mg amoxicillin, 62.5 mg potassium clavulanate

Storage: Keep liquid forms of this medication in the refrigerator. Discard unused liquid after 14 days. Store all forms in tightly closed containers.

Before Using This Drug, Tell Your Doctor: if you are allergic to penicillin or have a history of liver or kidney problems. Tell your doctor if you have mononucleosis. Tell your doctor about any drugs, prescription or nonprescription, you are taking and about any allergies you have or any family history of allergies.

This Drug Should Not Be Used If: you are allergic to any form of penicillin or have mononucleosis.

How to Use: Take Augmentin as directed by your doctor, usually every eight hours. This drug can be taken with or without food. If you are using the oral suspension, shake the bottle well before measuring the dose and use a medical teaspoon, not a kitchen spoon.

Time Required for Drug to Take Effect: usually two to five days, depending on the infection being treated. However, you should continue to take the medication for the full time your doctor has prescribed, even if you seem well; otherwise, the infection may return.

Missing a Dose: Take the missed dose immediately, but if it is almost time for the next dose, wait to take the next dose until about halfway through the regular interval between doses. For example, if you are to take a dose at 8:00 A.M., 4:00 P.M., and midnight, and you remember at 3:00 P.M. that you forgot the 8:00 A.M. dose, take the missed dose at 3:00 P.M. but wait until 8:00 P.M. to take the 4:00 P.M. dose. Then return to the regular schedule. Do not skip a dose or double the dose.

Symptoms of Overdose: possible severe and persistent nausea, vomiting, and/or diarrhea

Side Effects:

Minor and expected:
- diarrhea, nausea, vomiting, headache, stomach discomfort

Serious adverse reactions (CALL YOUR DOCTOR):
- hives, itching, or skin rash; difficult breathing; fever; joint pain; sore throat; dark-colored tongue; yellow-green stools; sores in the mouth; severe and persistent nausea, vomiting, and diarrhea

Effects of Long-Term Use: superinfection—a second infection in addition to the infection being treated. The superinfection is caused by bacteria and other organisms that are not susceptible to or affected by the drug being used to treat the original infection. Thus these organisms, which are normally too few in number to cause problems, grow unchecked and cause a second infection that may require treatment with a different drug

Habit-Forming Possibility: none

Precautions and Suggestions:

Foods and beverages:
- No restrictions.

Other medicines, prescription and nonprescription:
- Antacids and other antibiotics reduce the absorption and effect of Augmentin.
- Augmentin may also interact with the gout medication probenecid.

Other:
- If mild diarrhea is a side effect, ask your doctor if you can eat yogurt. The beneficial bacteria in yogurt replace the intestine's natural beneficial bacteria that have been reduced or eliminated by Augmentin
- This drug should be taken for the full length of time recommended by your doctor even if you seem to have recovered. Otherwise, the infection may return and be more difficult to treat the second time.
- Do not use the medication beyond the expiration date on the label. As a general rule of thumb, discard any unused liquid medication that has been refrigerated after 14 days.
- If you ever have any doubts about how you are reacting to a medicine, call your doctor.

Medical Tests:

- Your doctor may recommend tests during treatment with this drug, including blood counts and liver and kidney function tests, to monitor your progress.
- Any drug may affect the results and accuracy of a medical test. If a doctor recommends a medical or laboratory test for any condition, inform the doctor that you are taking Augmentin.

BACTRIM

Ingredient(s): trimethoprim and sulfamethoxazole

Equivalent Product(s): Bethaprim, Cotrim, Septra, Sulfatrim, trimethoprim and sulfamethoxazole (generic)

Used for: treatment of infections, especially in the urinary tract, middle ear, lungs, or intestines

Dosage Form and Strength: tablets—80 mg trimethoprim, 400 mg sulfamethoxazole; 160 mg trimethoprim, 800 mg sulfamethoxazole; oral suspension—40 mg trimethoprim, 200 mg sulfamethoxazole per 5 ml (1 medical teaspoon)

Storage: Store at room temperature.

Before Using This Drug, Tell Your Doctor: if you have liver or kidney disease, any vitamin deficiencies, severe allergies, bronchial asthma, diabetes, or glucose-6-phosphate dehydrogenase deficiency. Also tell your doctor about any other drugs, prescription or nonprescription, you are using.

This Drug Should Not Be Used If: you are allergic to its ingredients or to sulfa drugs or if you are anemic because of a vitamin deficiency. Bactrim should not be used to treat strep throat because it is not effective enough.

How to Use: Take each dose with a full glass of water. Take all the medication prescribed even if your symptoms disappear and you feel well. While taking this drug, you should drink plenty of water—at least eight glasses each day.

Time Required for Drug to Take Effect: five to 14 days

Missing a Dose: Take the missed dose immediately. If it is almost time for the next dose, take that next dose midway through the interval between doses. Then return to the regular schedule. Do not skip a dose.

Symptoms of Overdose: A maximum tolerated dose in humans is unknown. However, in studies in which animals were given large doses of the drug, they developed tremors or convulsions, slowed breathing, reduced activity, and loss of muscular coordination

Side Effects:

Minor and expected:
- abdominal pain, loss of appetite, nausea, diarrhea, dizziness, headache, vomiting, sensitivity to the sun, sore mouth

Serious adverse reactions (CALL YOUR DOCTOR):
- rash, mouth sores, unusual bleeding and bruising, sore throat, fever, paleness, skin discoloration, difficult urination, reduced urine output, breathing difficulties, fluid retention, itching (especially in genital and anal areas), convulsions, ringing in the ears, tingling in the hands or feet, weakness, blood disorders, muscle weakness, kidney disorders

Effects of Long-Term Use: possible reduction in the ability of the bone marrow, the soft connective tissue inside the bones, to do its job of manufacturing blood cells, thus leading to a deficiency of certain blood cells

Habit-Forming Possibility: none

Precautions and Suggestions:

Foods and beverages:
- No restrictions.

Other medicines, prescription and nonprescription:
- Bactrim may react with phenytoin (Dilantin), diuretics, gout drugs, oral diabetes medicines, oral anticoagulants, some cancer drugs, barbiturates, isoniazid, local anesthetics, methenamines, phenylbutazone, antibiotics (oxacillin, penicillins), and para-aminobenzoic acid (PABA) found in sunscreens.
- Tell your doctor about any drugs you are currently taking.

Other:
- This drug may cause you to be sensitive to the sun. Be sure you are not exposed to the sun or are protected by a sunscreen that does *not* contain PABA.

Medical Tests:

- Some doctors may suggest complete blood counts and liver and kidney tests to monitor your progress.
- Bactrim can interfere with the results of some blood and urine tests, including home urine test for glucose.
- Any drug may affect the results and accuracy of a medical test. If a doctor recommends a medical or laboratory test for any condition, inform the doctor that you are taking this drug.

CATAPRES

Ingredient(s): clonidine

Equivalent Product(s): none

Used for: treating high blood pressure

Dosage Form and Strength: tablets—0.1 mg, 0.2 mg, 0.3 mg

Storage: Store in a dry, tightly closed container.

Before Using This Drug, Tell Your Doctor: if you have a history of heart disease, angina, stroke, blood vessel disease, Raynaud's disease, kidney disease, eye disease, or mental depression. Also tell your doctor about any drugs, prescription or nonprescription, you are taking and about any allergies you have or any family history of allergies.

This Drug Should Not Be Used If: you are allergic to its ingredient. This drug should be used with caution by those with heart or blood vessel disease or kidney failure or by those who have had a recent heart attack.

How to Use: Take Catapres with food or water

Time Required for Drug to Take Effect: Blood pressure decreases within 30 to 60 minutes after a dose, and the maximum reduction occurs within two to four hours. The antihypertensive effect lasts about 12 to 24 hours.

Missing a Dose: Take the missed dose as soon as you remember unless it is close to your next regular dose. If that is the case, do not take the missed dose at all, but return to the regular dosing schedule. Do not double the dose.

Symptoms of Overdose: extreme drowsiness, slow and weak pulse, weakness, deep sleep, lowered body temperature, breathing problems, seizures, agitation, irritability, diarrhea, heartbeat irregularities

Side Effects:

Minor and expected:
- dry mouth and nose, drowsiness, sleepiness, constipation, headache, fatigue, loss of appetite

Serious adverse reactions (CALL YOUR DOCTOR):
- dizziness, nausea, vomiting, pain in salivary gland, weight gain, breast enlargement in men, vivid dreams, nightmares, sleeplessness, nervousness, restlessness, changes in behavior, anxiety, depression, rash, hives, itching, thinning hair, impotence, urination difficulty, burning eyes, paleness

Effects of Long-Term Use: weight gain caused by retention of fluid, temporary impotence. You may develop a tolerance to the effects of the drug, necessitating reevaluation of the dosage or therapy.

Habit-Forming Possibility: none

Precautions and Suggestions:

Foods and beverages:
- No food restrictions
- Avoid alcohol; Catapres can cause an increased sensitivity to alcohol.

Other medicines, prescription and nonprescription:

- Avoid cough, cold, allergy, and sinus medications while taking Catapres.
- Catapres may interact with sedatives, barbiturates, tranquilizers, sleeping aids, antihistamines, narcotics, pain relievers, and other drugs that depress the central nervous system.
- This drug also interacts with tricyclic antidepressants and the vasodilator tolazoline.
- Catapres may interact with other drugs for high blood pressure and with diuretics.

Other:

- Do not discontinue this medication abruptly. Sudden withdrawal can cause a rapid rise in blood pressure and possibly cause a severe and dangerous reaction. If you develop an illness that causes vomiting so that you cannot take this drug on a regular basis, tell your doctor.
- Hot weather, heat (as in a hot workplace), and fever accompanying illness can reduce blood pressure; you may have to have your doctor adjust your dosage if hot weather or fever affects you.
- If this drug makes you drowsy or dizzy, do not engage in activities that require alertness, such as driving a car or operating potentially dangerous machinery.
- This drug may cause painful numbing of hands and feet when they are exposed to extreme cold.
- Use caution with isometric exercises. Such exercises can raise blood pressure, and this drug can intensify the hypertensive response to these exercises.

Medical Tests:

- Your doctor may want to perform periodic eye examinations since some studies have documented changes in the eye in animals while taking this drug.
- If your doctor orders a Coombs test for anemia, tell him or her you are taking Catapres; this drug may cause weakly positive Coombs test results.
- This drug may affect the results of laboratory tests, especially blood tests and liver function tests.
- Any drug may affect the results and accuracy of a medical test. If a doctor recommends a medical or laboratory test for any condition, inform the doctor that you are taking this drug.

CECLOR

Ingredient(s): cefaclor

Equivalent Product(s): none

Used for: treatment of bacterial infections

Dosage Form and Strength: capsules—250 mg, 500 mg; oral suspension—125 mg per 5 ml, 250 mg per 5 ml

Storage: Store liquid in refrigerator. Discard unused portion after 14 days. Store capsules in dry, tightly closed containers at room temperature.

Before Using This Drug, Tell Your Doctor: if you are allergic to any antibiotics, especially cephalosporins and penicillin. Also tell your doctor if you have a history of kidney or liver problems, colitis, blood-clotting problems, or diabetes. Tell your doctor about any drugs, prescription or nonprescription, you are taking and about any allergies you have or any family history of allergies.

This Drug Should Not Be Used If: you are allergic to its ingredient.

How to Use: Take this drug at regularly spaced intervals around the clock. This drug can be taken with or without food, but if upset stomach occurs, take the dose with food. Take the capsule with a full glass of water. If you are using the oral suspension, shake it well before measuring the dose. Take either dosage form for the full time recommended even if you seem well.

Time Required for Drug to Take Effect: varies, depending on the infection being treated. Using the drug for two to five days is usually necessary to see if the drug is effective against the infection being treated.

Missing a Dose: Take the missed dose immediately. However, if it is almost time for your next dose, space the next dose about midway through the regular interval between doses. For example, if you are supposed to take a dose at 8:00 A.M., 4:00 P.M., and midnight, and you remember at 3:00 P.M. that you forgot the 8:00 A.M. dose, take the missed dose at 3:00 P.M. but wait until 8:00 P.M. to take the 4:00 P.M. dose. Then return to the regular schedule. Do not skip a dose or double the dose.

Symptoms of Overdose: abdominal cramping, nausea, vomiting, diarrhea

Side Effects:

Minor and expected:
- upset stomach, nausea, diarrhea, loss of appetite, headache, dizziness, fatigue, sores in the mouth

Serious adverse reactions (CALL YOUR DOCTOR):
- severe diarrhea, rash, fever, itching (especially in genital and anal areas), hives, joint pain, difficult breathing, sore throat, tingling in hands and feet

Effects of Long-Term Use: superinfection—that is, a second infection in addition to the infection being treated. A superinfection is caused by bacteria and other organisms that are not susceptible to or affected by the drug being used to treat the original infection. Thus, these organisms, which are normally too few in number to cause problems, grow unchecked and cause a second infection that may require treatment with a different drug.

Habit-Forming Possibility: none

Precautions and Suggestions:

Foods and beverages:
- There are no food restrictions, although Ceclor is more effective if taken one hour before or two hours after a meal. Nevertheless, it can be taken at any time.
- Ask your doctor if you can drink alcoholic beverages while taking Ceclor.

Other medicines, prescription and nonprescription:
- Ceclor interacts with other antibiotics, oral anticoagulants, probenecid gout medicine, and some diuretics. Tell your doctor if you are taking any other drugs.

Other:
- If mild diarrhea is a side effect, ask your doctor if you can eat yogurt. The beneficial bacteria in yogurt replace the intestine's natural beneficial bacteria that have been reduced or eliminated by Ceclor.

Medical Tests:

- Ceclor may interfere with the results of some blood and urine tests, including some home tests for glucose.
- If Ceclor is being used to treat a sexually transmitted disease, your doctor may require diagnostic tests for up to three months.
- Any drug may affect the results and accuracy of a medical test. If a doctor recommends a medical or laboratory test for any condition, inform the doctor that you are taking this drug.

CLINORIL

Ingredient(s): sulindac

Equivalent Product(s): none

Used for: relief of symptoms of arthritis, bursitis, gout, and ankylosing spondylitis

Dosage Form and Strength: tablets—150 mg, 200 mg

Storage: Store in a dry, tightly closed container.

Before Using This Drug, Tell Your Doctor: if you have liver or kidney disease, stomach or intestinal problems including ulcers, bleeding problems, heart disease, high blood pressure, anemia, diabetes, epilepsy, parkinsonism, or a history of sensitivity to aspirin. Tell your doctor about any drugs, prescription or nonprescription, that you are taking and about any allergies you have, especially to aspirin, sulindac, ibuprofen, fenoprofen, naproxen, naproxen sodium, indomethacin, tolmetin, zomepirac, mefenamic acid, meclofenamate, or piroxicam. Tell your doctor about any family history of allergies.

This Drug Should Not Be Used If: you are allergic to aspirin or any nonsteroidal anti-inflammatory drug (listed at the end of the preceding paragraph), including the ingredient in this medication. This drug should be used with caution by those who have liver or kidney disease, bleeding disorders, an active ulcer, or ulcerative colitis.

How to Use: It is preferable to take this drug on an empty stomach 30 to 60 minutes before meals or two hours after a meal. However, your doctor may recommend you take it with food, especially if stomach upset occurs.

Time Required for Drug to Take Effect: one to two hours, although it may take about seven days before significant improvement is noticeable

Missing a Dose: Take the missed dose as soon as you remember, unless it is nearly time for your next dose. In that case, omit the missed dose and return to your regular dosing schedule. Do not double the next dose.

Symptoms of Overdose: stomach upset, nausea, vomiting, diarrhea

Side Effects:

Minor and expected:
- mild stomach upset and/or cramping, drowsiness, heartburn, bloating, gas, dry mouth, loss of appetite, dizziness, headache, constipation, mild diarrhea, nervousness

Serious adverse reactions (CALL YOUR DOCTOR):
- severe stomach upset, nausea, vomiting, or diarrhea; abdominal pain; black, tarry stools; rectal bleeding; nosebleeds; mouth sores; severe headache; yellowish discoloration of skin and eyes; tremor; convulsions; muscle pain or weakness; fatigue; lethargy; numbness, prickling, tingling; nerve disorders; sleepiness or sleeplessness; depression; confusion; behavior changes; fall or rise in blood pressure; changes in heartbeat; fluid retention; chest pain; blood in urine; problems with urination; blood disorders; purplish discoloration of skin; bruising; anemia; changes in vision; irritated eyes; sensitivity to light; loss of color vision (reversible when drug is stopped); ringing in the ears; hearing loss; ear pain; stuffy nose; changes in taste; breathing difficulty; rash; itching; baldness; aggravation of epilepsy and parkinsonism; changes in blood sugar levels and increased need for insulin in diabetics; increased blood potassium levels; flushing or sweating; menstrual disorders; vaginal bleeding; vaginal infection; unexplained sore throat and fever; chills; thirst; fainting; sore tongue; breast changes in men and women

Effects of Long-Term Use: Eye problems have been reported with the use of similar drugs but have not been proven with Clinoril.

Habit-Forming Possibility: none

Precautions and Suggestions:

Foods and beverages:
- No food restrictions.
- Consult your doctor before consuming alcoholic beverages with this drug.

Other medicines, prescription and nonprescription:
- Avoid aspirin while using this drug.
- Avoid antacids containing large amounts of sodium.
- Clinoril may interact with anticonvulsants, phenobarbital, sulfa drugs, diuretics, beta blockers, diabetes medications, anticoagulant drugs, other anti-inflammatory drugs, other arthritis or gout medications, or aspirin.

Other:
- If this drug causes drowsiness, dizziness, or blurred vision, do not engage in activities that require alertness, such as driving or operating potentially dangerous machinery.
- Because of its anti-inflammatory and fever-reducing qualities, this drug may mask the development of an infection. If you suspect an infection, call your doctor.

- Before any medical treatment, including dental treatment, tell your health-care provider that you are taking this drug.

Medical Tests:

- Your doctor may want to conduct periodic liver and kidney function tests, blood tests, and eye examinations.
- Clinoril may interfere with the results of some laboratory tests; be certain to remind your doctor or lab technician that you are taking Clinoril when you are being tested.

CODEINE (GENERIC)

Ingredient(s): codeine

Equivalent Product(s): Codeine is available as a single drug in generic form only. However, many brand-name combination products contain codeine.

Used for: relief of mild to moderate pain and for dry cough

Dosage Form and Strength: tablets—15 mg, 30 mg, 60 mg; soluble tablets—15 mg, 30 mg, 60 mg

Storage: Store in a dry, tightly closed container away from light.

Before Using This Drug, Tell Your Doctor: if you have a history of liver, kidney, heart, or thyroid conditions; a recent head injury; asthma or any lung disorder; or epilepsy or other convulsive disorder. Tell your doctor if you have a history of alcoholism, delirium tremens, cerebral arteriosclerosis, Addison's disease, curvature of the spine (kyphoscoliosis), enlarged prostate, narrowing of the urethra, psychosis, or severe central nervous system depression. Also, tell your doctor about any drugs, prescription or nonprescription, you are taking and about any allergies you have or any family history of allergies.

This Drug Should Not Be Used If: you are allergic to it. This drug is not recommended for use during a bout of diarrhea caused by poisoning until the poison is eliminated from the body. This drug should be used with caution for anyone in a coma.

How to Use: Take this medication with food or milk to prevent stomach upset.

Time Required for Drug to Take Effect: 15 to 30 minutes

Missing a Dose: Take the missed dose as soon as possible unless it is almost time for the next dose. In this case, do not take the missed dose, but return to the regular schedule. Never double the dose.

Symptoms of Overdose: severe drowsiness, nausea, vomiting, restlessness, excitability, deep sleep, convulsions, clammy skin, shallow breathing, constricted pupils, limpness

Side Effects:

Minor and expected:
- drowsiness, dry mouth, constipation, light-headedness

Serious adverse reactions (CALL YOUR DOCTOR):
- rash, hives, itching, nausea, vomiting, dizziness, blurred vision, sweating, headache, sleeplessness, mood changes, tremors, uncoordinated muscles, difficulty in breathing, fear, anxiety, confusion, agitation

Effects of Long-Term Use: physical and psychological dependence

Habit-Forming Possibility: strong. This drug can lead to dependence when used in large doses and/or for long periods of time.

Precautions and Suggestions:

Foods and beverages:
- No food restrictions.
- Avoid alcohol. Even if you do not drink alcoholic beverages, make sure that you are not taking another medication containing alcohol.

Other medicines, prescription and nonprescription:
- Codeine may interact with other narcotics, sedatives, tranquilizers, anesthetics, barbiturates, antihistamines, monoamineoxidase inhibitors, painkillers, and antidepressants.
- Codeine interacts with the drug chlodiazepoxide (Librium).
- Aspirin and the antibiotic chloramphenicol increase the painkilling action of codeine.
- There have been reports of reactions when narcotics are taken at the same time as cimetidine (Tagamet), although no clear-cut cause-and-effect relationship has been established.

Other:
- If this drug causes you to become drowsy, do not engage in activities that require alertness.
- If it has been necessary to take this medication for a long period of time, ask your doctor how to reduce the dosage and eventually stop taking the drug. This drug is recommended only for short-term use.

Medical Tests:

- Codeine may interfere with liver tests.

- Any drug may affect the results and accuracy of a medical test. If a doctor recommends a medical or laboratory test for any condition, inform the doctor that you are taking this drug.

CORGARD

Ingredient(s): nadolol

Equivalent Product(s): none

Used for: managing angina and high blood pressure

Dosage Form and Strength: tablets—40 mg, 80 mg, 120 mg, 160 mg

Storage: Store in a tightly closed container at room temperature away from light, heat, and moisture.

Before Using This Drug, Tell Your Doctor: if you have asthma or any respiratory problems, including chronic obstructive pulmonary disease, bronchitis, or emphysema; a history of heart disease; congestive heart failure; poor circulation in fingers and toes; hypoglycemia; diabetes; overactive thyroid gland; or kidney or liver disease. Tell your doctor about any drugs, prescription or nonprescription, you are taking and about any allergies you have or any family history of allergies.

This Drug Should Not Be Used If: you are allergic to its ingredient or have a slow heartbeat, heart block greater than first degree, cardiogenic shock, heart failure (unless it results from a condition treatable by this type of drug), bronchial asthma, bronchospasm (including that associated with respiratory allergies like hay fever), or severe chronic obstructive pulmonary disease.

How to Use: This drug may be taken without regard to meals. Follow your doctor's advice about when to take the drug. Try to take the drug at the same time every day. Do not stop taking the drug abruptly unless your doctor instructs you to do so.

Time Required for Drug to Take Effect: one hour, reaching a peak in three to four hours, and persisting for 24 hours. Consistent use for several weeks may be necessary to determine Corgard's effectiveness in treating your condition.

Missing a Dose: Take the missed dose as soon as you remember unless you are due to take the next scheduled dose within eight hours if you take the drug once a day, or within four hours if you take the drug more than once a day. In that case, omit the missed dose and maintain your regular schedule. Do not double the next dose.

Symptoms of Overdose: slow and/or weak pulse, weakness, dizziness on standing up, fainting, loss of consciousness, delirium, seizures, difficult or slowed breathing, bronchospasm, clammy skin

Side Effects:

Minor and expected:
- drowsiness, dry mouth, cold hands and feet, fatigue

Serious adverse reactions (CALL YOUR DOCTOR):
- light-headedness in upright position, sore throat, fever, breathing difficulties, night cough, wheezing, nasal stuffiness, chest pain, slow pulse (less than 60 beats per minute), retention of fluids, worsening of angina or asthma, wheezing, heartbeat irregularities, dizziness, fainting, depression, lethargy, sleeplessness, anxiety, nervousness, nightmares or odd dreams, confusion, behavior changes, hallucinations, slurred speech, ringing in the ears, headache, short-term memory loss, numbness or tingling of fingers and toes, reduced sexual interest and/or ability, abdominal pain or cramping, nausea, vomiting, constipation, diarrhea, loss of appetite, urination difficulties and/or frequency, bruising, eye discomfort, dry and burning eyes, blurred vision, rash, itching, skin irritation, dry skin, sweating, changes in skin color, reversible baldness, joint pain, muscle cramps and pain

Effects of Long-Term Use: Long-term use in high doses may lead to reduced strength of heart muscle, which may increase the risk of heart failure.

Habit-Forming Possibility: none

Precautions and Suggestions:

Foods and beverages:
- No food restrictions.
- Consult your doctor before drinking alcoholic beverages because alcohol may increase the action of Corgard.

Other medicines, prescription and nonprescription:
- Corgard may interact with anesthetics and should be discontinued gradually before any surgery. Be certain your doctor, surgeon, and/or dentist knows you are taking this drug before any surgical procedure is begun.
- Nicotine in tobacco may decrease the effectiveness of this drug. Ask your doctor about smoking while taking this drug.
- Corgard may increase the effects of other high blood pressure medications, insulin and oral antidiabetes drugs, barbiturates, narcotics, and reserpine.

- Corgard may decrease the effects of aspirin, cortisone, and other anti-inflammatory drugs. Corgard also decreases the effects of antihistamines used to treat allergies.
- Corgard also may interact with digitalis, digoxin, verapamil (Isoptin), nifedipine (Procardia), diltiazem, quinidine, phenytoin (Dilantin), chlorpromazine, phenothiazines, monoamine oxidase inhibitors, cimetidine (Tagamet), oral contraceptives, furosemide (Lasix), hydralazine, rifampin, phenobarbital, indomethacin, prazosin, isoproterenol, norepinephrine, dopamine, dobutamine, theophylline and other bronchodilators, and clonidine.

Other:
- Do not stop taking this drug abruptly unless your doctor instructs you to do so. This drug must be discontinued gradually.
- If this drug makes you dizzy or drowsy, do not engage in activities that require alertness, such as driving a car or operating potentially dangerous machinery.
- This drug may hide the signs of impending hypoglycemia and change the blood sugar levels in diabetics. If you are diabetic, work with your doctor to adjust dosages of your diabetes medications to compensate for this drug.
- Do not take any nonprescription products for cough, cold, allergy, weight control, or sinus problems without calling your doctor first.

Medical Tests:
- This drug may interfere with glucose and insulin tolerance tests.
- If you are taking Corgard on a long-term basis, your doctor may want to perform blood tests to monitor your progress.
- Your doctor may ask you to take your pulse each day; if it drops below 60 beats per minute, call your doctor.
- Any drug may affect the results and accuracy of a medical test. If a doctor recommends a medical or laboratory test for any condition, inform the doctor that you are taking this drug.

COUMADIN

Ingredient(s): warfarin sodium

Equivalent Product(s): Coufarin, Panwarfin, warfarin sodium (generic)

Used for: prevention and treatment of blood clot formation

Dosage Form and Strength: tablets—2 mg, 2.5 mg, 5 mg, 7.5 mg, 10 mg

Storage: Store in tightly closed container away from light.

Before Using This Drug, Tell Your Doctor: if you have bleeding tendencies or disorders, hemophilia, polycythemia vera, thrombocytopenic purpura, leukemia, gastrointestinal bleeding, ulcers, ulcerative colitis, kidney or liver disease, diverticulitis, blood disorders, high blood pressure, heart or blood vessel disease, aneurysm, widespread arthritis, cancer, thyroid disorders, pancreas disorder, an infection, diet deficiencies, diabetes, tuberculosis, or a high cholesterol count. Tell your doctor if you have just undergone or are about to undergo a surgical procedure, either medical or dental. Tell your doctor about any diagnostic procedures you have had recently or will be undergoing. Tell your doctor about any recent injuries. Tell your doctor about any drugs, prescription or nonprescription, you are taking and about any allergies you have or any family history of allergies.

This Drug Should Not Be Used If: you have bleeding tendencies or disorders, hemophilia, thrombocytopenic purpura, leukemia, ulcers, gastrointestinal bleeding, aneurysm, ascorbic acid deficiency, kidney infection, suspected cerebrovascular bleeding, diverticulitis, blood disorders, uncontrolled high blood pressure, liver disease, some heart disorders (pericardial effusion, bacterial endocarditis), ulcerative colitis, internal cancer, widespread arthritis, polycythemia vera, severe injury, diet deficiencies, blood vessel disorders, some allergies, severe diabetes, or an indwelling catheter. This drug should not be used if you recently had surgery or are planning surgery, and it should not be used if you are having diagnostic or therapeutic procedures that may potentially lead to uncontrolled bleeding. This drug is also contraindicated for those with infections requiring antibiotic therapy that may alter the internal intestinal environment and for those who have an allergy to its ingredient.

How to Use: Take with a full glass of water at the times recommended by your doctor. Try to take the medicine at the same time every day.

Time Required for Drug to Take Effect: The drug's action begins in 24 to 36 hours and is effective within 36 to 72 hours. You may have to take the drug on a continuous basis for up to two weeks while testing blood-clotting time to help your doctor determine the necessary maintenance dose.

Missing a Dose: Take the missed dose as soon as you remember unless it is almost time for the next dose. In that case, do not take the missed dose, but return to your regular schedule. Tell your doctor about any doses you miss.

Symptoms of Overdose: prolonged bleeding from shaving nicks or other minor injuries, bleeding gums, bruising, blood spots in white of eye, nosebleeds, vomiting of blood, blood in urine or stool

Side Effects:

Minor and expected:
- minor bleeding from nicks or scratches (an electric razor is recommended)

Serious adverse reactions (CALL YOUR DOCTOR):
- unexplained or excessive bleeding or bruising of the skin, gums, or nose; blood in vomit, urine, or stool; rash; fatigue; chills; fever; sore throat; yellowish discoloration of skin or white of eyes; hair loss; hives; itching; nausea; vomiting; loss of appetite; abdominal cramps; diarrhea; mouth sores; sustained penile erection

Effects of Long-Term Use: none known

Habit-Forming Possibility: none

Precautions and Suggestions:

Foods and beverages:
- Avoid large amounts of green, leafy vegetables and alcohol.
- Do not change your diet or eating habits without consulting your doctor.

Other medicines, prescription and nonprescription:
- *Do not* take any other medication, prescription or nonprescription, without talking to your doctor.
- *Do not* take aspirin or any products containing aspirin or salicylates while taking Coumadin.
- The effects of Coumadin may be increased by oral antibiotics, salicylates, sulfa drugs, oral diabetes drugs, triclofos, chloral hydrate, clofibrate, chloramphenicol, allopurinol, disulfiram, metronidazole, cimetidine, thyroid drugs, anabolic steroids, quinidine, glucagon, danazol, and sulindac.
- An increased tendency to bleed may occur if Coumadin is taken with aspirin or salicylates, sulfinpyrazone, phenylbutazone, oxyphenbutazone, indomethacin, dipyridamole, quinidine, quinine, antimetabolites, alkylating agents, adrenal corticosteroids, and potassium products.
- The effects of Coumadin may be decreased by barbiturates, glutethimide, ethchlorvynol, griseofulvin, phenytoin, carbamazepine, rifampin, estrogens, vitamin K, cholestyramine, colestipol, and diuretics.

- Coumadin also interacts with streptokinase, urokinase, antihistamines, other oral anticoagulants, sedatives and tranquilizers, antihypertension drugs, acetaminophen, antidepressants, tuberculosis drugs, nonsteroid anti-inflammatory drugs, methylphenidate, urinary anti-infectives, gout medicines, and digitalis preparations.

Other:
- Avoid contact sports or any activity that may lead to an injury.
- Some forms of this drug contain a dye called *tartrazine* that may cause allergic reactions (including bronchial asthma). This often occurs in people who are sensitive to aspirin.
- This drug may cause a red-orange discoloration of the urine. You can determine that this discoloration is not blood by adding an acid such as vinegar to the urine. If the discoloration disappears with the addition of vinegar, it is not being caused by blood.
- Be certain to tell your doctor, surgeon, or dentist that you are taking Coumadin before any surgery or treatment.
- Do not stop taking this drug suddenly and do not change dosage without your doctor's instructions.
- Carry an identification card that states you are taking Coumadin.
- The effects of this drug can last a few days after discontinuation, so you should be careful about injury after stopping this drug.

Medical Tests:

- You doctor will want to perform blood tests to determine blood-clotting time, especially when you start using this drug, but also on a periodic and regular basis.
- Your doctor may want to perform liver function tests and urinalyses while you are taking Coumadin.
- Coumadin may interfere with the results of some urine tests.
- Most acute illnesses can cause changes in the effect of Coumadin; therefore, during such an illness testing may be required to determine how this drug is working.
- Any drug may affect the results and accuracy of a medical test. If a doctor recommends a medical or laboratory test for any condition, inform the doctor that you are taking this drug.

CROMOLYN SODIUM (GENERIC)

Ingredient(s): cromolyn sodium (disodium cromoglycate)
Equivalent Product(s): Intal, Nasalcrom

Used for: prevention of attacks of severe bronchial asthma and prevention and treatment of runny nose due to an allergy. This drug will not relieve an asthma attack once it has begun; cromolyn is strictly a preventive medication.

Dosage Form and Strength: capsules for inhalation only—20 mg; solution for spray device—20 mg per 2 ml ampule; nasal solution—40 mg per ml (each spray delivers 5.2 mg)

Storage: Store in a dry, tightly closed container in a cool, dark place. Do not refrigerate. Do not handle the inhaler or capsules with wet hands.

Before Using This Drug, Tell Your Doctor: if you have a history of liver or kidney disease. Also tell your doctor about any drugs, prescription or nonprescription, that you are taking (especially other drugs for asthma) and about any allergies you have or any family history of allergies.

This Drug Should Not Be Used If: you have an allergy to its ingredient.

How to Use: The capsules are to be inhaled, not taken by mouth. Ask your doctor to explain and demonstrate how to inhale the capsules. Also, ask your pharmacist to include a sheet of patient instructions with the prescription. Be certain you understand how to use this form of the medication before you take it. The spray solution should be administered from a power-operated sprayer equipped with a face mask. A hand-operated sprayer is not acceptable. This too should be inhaled. Ask your doctor to show you how to use this product. After using either the capsules or the spray inhaler, rinse your mouth and throat with water to prevent irritation. The nasal solution should be sprayed once into each nostril at regular intervals during the day. You should clear out your nose before using the spray and should inhale through the nose while spraying the solution. This solution should be administered with a metered spray device that should be replaced every six months. Ask your doctor to explain how to use this product.

Time Required for Drug to Take Effect: two to four weeks

Missing a Dose: Try not to miss a dose; this medication is effective only if taken at regular intervals. If you do forget, take the missed dose immediately. If it is almost time for the next dose, space that next dose midway through the regular intervals between doses. Then return to your regular schedule. For example, if you are to take a dose at 8:00 A.M., noon, 4:00 P.M., and 8:00 P.M., and you remember at 7:00 P.M. that you forgot the 4:00 P.M. dose, take the missed dose at 7:00 P.M. but wait until 9:30 or 10:00 P.M. to take the 8:00 P.M. dose. Do not skip a dose or double a dose.

Symptoms of Overdose: none reported

Side Effects:

Minor and expected:
- mild cough, throat irritation, or hoarseness; sneezing; nasal burning and stinging

Serious adverse reactions (CALL YOUR DOCTOR):
- rash, spasm of bronchial tubes with shortness of breath, severe cough, nosebleed, abdominal pain, nausea, headache, drowsiness, dizziness, pain and swelling in joints, difficult urination

Effects of Long-Term Use: allergic reaction of lung tissue, leading to a condition resembling pneumonia

Habit-Forming Possibility: none

Precautions and Suggestions:

Foods and beverages:
- There are no specific restrictions except to avoid foods to which you are allergic.

Other medicines, prescription and nonprescription:
- Cromolyn may interact with the bronchodilator isoproterenol. Tell your doctor if you are using a bronchodilator.
- The use of cromolyn may make it possible to reduce or discontinue cortisone or steroid drugs you may be taking for asthma. Do not adjust the doses yourself, but discuss this with your doctor.

Other:
- Do not stop taking cromolyn abruptly; this may trigger a return of an asthma attack.
- Do not swallow the capsule. If you do accidentally swallow the capsule, there will be no ill effects, but there will also be no beneficial effects.
- Do not change recommended dosages yourself. Sometimes cromolyn is effective enough that a person believes the dosage can be reduced. This may trigger an asthma attack. Always talk with your doctor before changing a drug's dosage.

Medical Tests:

- Your doctor may suggest tests to examine your lungs if you develop symptoms suggesting an allergic reaction of lung tissue to the drug. Such a reaction is rare.
- Any drug may affect the results and accuracy of a medical test. If a doctor recommends a medical or laboratory test for any condition, inform the doctor that you are taking this drug.

DALMANE

Ingredient(s): flurazepam hydrochloride

Equivalent Product(s): flurazepam hydrochloride (generic)

Used for: insomnia, including difficulty in falling asleep, awaking frequently during the night, and early morning wakefulness

Dosage Form and Strength: capsules—15 mg, 30 mg

Storage: Store in tightly closed container away from light and excessive heat.

Before Using This Drug, Tell Your Doctor: if you have a history of liver or kidney disease, chronic lung problems, epilepsy, acute intermittent porphyria, or a history of drug dependence. Tell your doctor about any drugs, prescription or nonprescription, you are taking and about any allergies you have or any family history of allergy.

This Drug Should Not Be Used If: you are allergic to its ingredient.

How to Use: Take Dalmane 30 minutes to an hour before bedtime with food or a full glass of water.

Time Required for Drug to Take Effect: 30 to 60 minutes

Missing a Dose: Take the missed dose only if you remember within an hour of the usual time. Otherwise, omit the missed dose. Do not double the next dose.

Symptoms of Overdose: extreme drowsiness or weakness, difficulty in walking and standing, deep sleep, confusion, loss of consciousness

Side Effects:

Minor and expected:
- drowsiness (after a night's sleep), light-headedness, dizziness, heartburn, upset stomach

Serious adverse reactions (CALL YOUR DOCTOR):
- staggering, falling, extreme sleepiness, nervousness, talkativeness, headache, fear, irritability, confusion, loss of consciousness, nausea, vomiting, diarrhea, constipation, abdominal pain, weakness, heartbeat irregularities, chest pain, joint pain, changes in urination habits, sweating, flushes, blurred vision, burning eyes, faintness, shortness of breath, itching, rash, dry mouth, bitter taste, excessive salivation, loss of appetite, yellowish discoloration of the skin and whites of eyes, depression, euphoria, slurred speech, restlessness, hallucinations, excitement, stimulation

Effects of Long-Term Use: This drug is not recommended for long-term use because of the possibility of drug dependence and the possibility of the drug's affecting liver function.

Habit-Forming Possibility: Dalmane may lead to physical and psychological dependence if taken in large doses for long periods of time.

Precautions and Suggestions:

Foods and beverages:
- There are no food restrictions, but avoid alcohol while taking Dalmane.
- Drinks with caffeine (coffee, tea, cola) can decrease the effectiveness of Dalmane.

Other medicines, prescription and nonprescription:
- Dalmane may interact with antihistamines and other cold or allergy preparations, anticonvulsants, antidepressants, tranquilizers, other sleep medications, narcotics, barbiturates, painkillers, narcotics, levodopa, antacids, lithium, cimetidine, disulfiram, rifampin, or tuberculosis medicine.

Other:
- Do not stop taking this drug abruptly after prolonged use. Ask your doctor how to discontinue taking the drug gradually.
- This drug tends to accumulate in the body. It is often recommended that it not be taken for more than two nights in a row, especially by an older person. Some doctors also think this drug should be used with great caution by anyone over 65 years of age.
- Do not engage in activities that require alertness, such as driving a car or operating potentially dangerous machinery.

Medical Tests:

- Your doctor may want to perform periodic blood tests as well as liver and kidney function tests to monitor your progress on this drug if you take it for a prolonged period of time.
- Dalmane can affect the results of some laboratory tests.
- Any drug may affect the results and accuracy of a medical test. If a doctor recommends a medical or laboratory test for any condition, inform the doctor that you are taking this drug.

DARVOCET-N

Ingredient(s): propoxyphene napsylate, acetaminophen

Equivalent Product(s): Propacet 100

Used for: treatment of mild to moderate pain

Dosage Form and Strength: tablets—50 mg propoxyphene napsylate and 325 mg acetaminophen (called Darvocet-N 50 Tablets), 100 mg propoxyphene and 650 mg acetaminophen (called Darvocet-N 100 Tablets)

Storage: Store in a tightly closed container away from light.

Before Using This Drug, Tell Your Doctor: if you have a history of depression, suicide thoughts, drug dependence, liver disease, kidney disease, blood disorders, heart or lung disease, or G6PD deficiency. Tell your doctor about any drugs, prescription or nonprescription, you are taking and about any allergies you have or any family history of allergies.

This Drug Should Not Be Used If: you are allergic to either of its ingredients. This drug should not be used by those who are prone to drug dependence or who are suicidal.

How to Use: Take Darvocet-N with food or a glass of water. It is most effective if taken when pain begins rather than when it becomes severe.

Time Required for Drug to Take Effect: 30 minutes to two hours

Missing a Dose: Take the missed dose as soon as you remember unless it is almost time for the next dose. In that case, do not take the missed dose, but return to your regular schedule. *Do not* double the next dose.

Symptoms of Overdose: extreme drowsiness progressing to stupor, loss of consciousness, convulsions, slowed or difficult breathing, heartbeat irregularities, dilated pupils, severe nausea and vomiting, abdominal pain, chills, extreme drowsiness

Side Effects:

Minor and expected:
- dizziness, sleepiness, drowsiness, fatigue

Serious adverse reactions (CALL YOUR DOCTOR):
- nausea, vomiting, chills, headache, constipation, abdominal pain, rash, weakness, false sense of well-being, vision problems, depression without apparent cause, convulsions, difficult breathing, heartbeat irregularities, dilated pupils, yellowish discoloration of skin and whites of eyes, excitement, agitation, sleeplessness, diarrhea, unexplained sore throat and fever, abnormal bleeding or bruising, ringing in the ears, confusion, slurred speech, falling

Effects of Long-Term Use: possible physical and psychological dependence; possible development of anemia

Habit-Forming Possibility: possible physical and psychological dependence if taken in large doses for a prolonged period of time

Precautions and Suggestions:

Foods and beverages:
- No food restrictions.
- *Avoid* alcohol.
- Beverages with caffeine (coffee, tea, cola, cocoa) may increase the effects of this drug.

Other medicines, prescription and nonprescription:
- Darvocet-N interacts with sedatives, antidepressants, tranquilizers, muscle relaxants, barbiturates, phenobarbital, warfarin, carbamazepine, cold and allergy preparations, aspirin, narcotics, orphenadrine, and painkillers.
- Cigarette smoking may affect the action of Darvocet-N.

Other:
- If this drug makes you dizzy or drowsy, do not engage in activities that require alertness, such as driving a car or operating potentially dangerous equipment.
- Do not take this drug in larger doses than prescribed.

Medical Tests:

- This drug can interfere with the results of some urine tests.
- Any drug may affect the results and accuracy of a medical test. If a doctor recommends a medical or laboratory test for any condition, inform the doctor that you are taking this drug.

DIABINESE

Ingredient(s): chlorpropamide

Equivalent Product(s): chlorpropamide (generic)

Used for: treatment of non-insulin-dependent diabetes that cannot be controlled by diet alone

Dosage Form and Strength: tablets—100 mg, 250 mg

Storage: Store in a tightly closed container.

Before Using This Drug, Tell Your Doctor: if you have a history of liver, kidney, thyroid, or endocrine disorders; heart disease; adrenal or pituitary gland insufficiency; ulcer; porphyria; or difficulty controlling your diabetes (brittle type). Tell your doctor about any drugs, prescription or nonprescription, you are taking and about any allergies you have or any family history of allergies.

This Drug Should Not Be Used If: you are allergic to its ingredient or to any other oral antidiabetes drug. This drug should not be used if you have serious liver, kidney, thyroid, or hormonal disorders. This drug should not be used by persons who have uremia, severe infections or injuries; who are undergoing major surgery; or who have severe diabetic reactions.

How to Use: Take with food, which must be an approved part of your diabetic diet. Take Diabinese at the precise times your doctor has prescribed.

Time Required for Drug to Take Effect: two to four hours. You may have to use the drug for one to two weeks to determine if it is controlling your diabetes effectively.

Missing a Dose: Take the missed dose as soon as you remember unless it is almost time for the next dose. In that case, do not take the missed dose, but return to your regular dosing schedule. Do not double the next dose. Call your doctor if you experience effects of missing a dose.

Symptoms of Overdose: hunger, nausea, tingling in lips and tongue, lethargy, confusion, yawning, agitation, nervousness, heartbeat irregularities, sweating, tremor, convulsions, stupor, loss of consciousness

Side Effects:

Minor and expected:
- headache, loss of appetite, nausea, vomiting, stomach discomfort, heartburn, weakness

Serious adverse reactions (CALL YOUR DOCTOR):
- fatigue, excessive hunger, profuse sweating, numbness in arms and legs, excessive thirst or urination, sugar or ketones in urine, rash, itching, hives, redness of skin, sensitivity to light, skin eruptions, yellowish discoloration of the skin, fluid retention, tingling in lips and tongue, lethargy, confusion, yawning, nervousness, heartbeat irregularities, sweating, tremor, convulsions, stupor, loss of consciousness, fever, sore throat, unusual bleeding or bruising, dark urine, light-colored stools

Effects of Long-Term Use: This drug has been associated with increased heart and blood vessel disease when compared to diet alone or diet and insulin as diabetes treatment. Discuss this risk with your doctor. This drug may also impair function of the thyroid gland if used for a prolonged time.

Habit-Forming Possibility: none

Precautions and Suggestions:

Foods and beverages:
- Your doctor will want you to maintain a strict diet to control your blood sugar. He or she will instruct you about your diet, exercise program, hygiene, and preventive health practices.
- Avoid alcohol; Diabinese can cause a reaction to alcohol similar to the reaction of Antabuse.

Other medicines, prescription and nonprescription:
- Diabinese's action can be increased or prolonged—therefore increasing the risk of hypoglycemia—by insulin, phenformin, sulfa drugs, chloramphenicol, fenfluramine, oxyphenbutazone, phenylbutazone, aspirin and other salicylates, nonsteroidal anti-inflammatory drugs, sulfinpyrazone, probenecid, monoamine oxidase inhibitors, clofibrate, and dicumarol.
- Diabinese's action can be decreased by beta-adrenergic blocking drugs.
- This drug also interacts with diazoxide and rifampin.
- Drugs that tend to cause high blood sugar and therefore loss of control of diabetes include diuretics, corticosteroids, phenothiazines, thyroid drugs, estrogens, phenytoin, nicotinic acid, cold and allergy products, bronchodilators, calcium channel blockers, and isoniazid.

Other:
- Do not discontinue use of the drug without your doctor's authorization.

- Test urine and blood for glucose on a regular basis as recommended by your doctor.
- Infections, illnesses, or injuries may require a change in your diabetes treatment, including using insulin instead of Diabinese. Inform your doctor if any of these circumstances occur.
- Use caution when exposed to sunlight; this drug can make you more sensitive to sunlight.

Medical Tests:

- Your doctor may want to perform blood counts, liver and thyroid function tests, and periodic heart and blood vessel examinations to monitor your progress while you take this drug.
- Any drug may affect the results and accuracy of a medical test. If a doctor recommends a medical or laboratory test for any condition, inform the doctor that you are taking this drug.

DILANTIN

Ingredient(s): phenytoin

Equivalent Product(s): none

Used for: control of epileptic seizures

Dosage Form and Strength: chewable tablets (Infatab)—50 mg; oral suspension—30 mg and 125 mg per 5 ml

Storage: Store at room temperature.

Before Using This Drug, Tell Your Doctor: if you have a history of liver, kidney, or heart disease; diabetes; low blood pressure; or bone disorders. Also, tell your doctor about any medications, OTC or prescription, you are taking; this includes aspirin and aspirin products, antibiotics, sulfa drugs, antacids, steroid drugs, some antidepressants, and other anticonvulsants. Be certain to tell your doctor about any allergies you have or any family history of allergies.

This Drug Should Not Be Used If: you are allergic to its ingredient.

How to Use: Take this drug with food to minimize stomach upset and to improve absorption. Shake the oral suspension well and measure in a medical teaspoon or dropper.

Time Required for Drug to Take Effect: It generally takes one to two weeks for the blood levels to stabilize.

Missing a Dose: Take the missed dose as soon as you remember unless it is almost time for the next dose, in which case you should eliminate the missed dose and return to the regular dosing schedule. Do not double the next dose. Call your doctor if you have a seizure as a result of missing a dose.

Symptoms of Overdose: constant involuntary movements of the eyeball, muscular incoordination, difficulty in moving joints, loss of consciousness

Side Effects:

Minor and expected:
- nausea, vomiting, diarrhea, constipation, drowsiness, dizziness, nervousness, insomnia, fatigue, irritability, headache, muscle twitching, tender gums, overgrowth of gum tissue, reddish or light brown urine color, blurred vision

Serious adverse reactions (CALL YOUR DOCTOR):
- rash, swollen glands, severe nausea or vomiting, joint pain, yellow discoloration of the skin, bleeding gums, sore throat, unexplained fever, unusual bleeding or bruising, persistent headache, chest pain, heartbeat irregularities, confusion, slurred speech, mouth sores, edema, loss of hair, weight gain, numbness

Effects of Long-Term Use: disorders of immune system, malignancies

Habit-Forming Possibility: none

Precautions and Suggestions:

Foods and beverages:
- No restrictions on food.
- Avoid alcoholic beverages.

Other medicines, prescription and nonprescription:
- This drug may interact with aspirin, aspirin products, some antibiotics, antidepressants, dopamine, valproic acid, phenacemide, diabetes drugs, and other anticonvulsants.
- Drugs that increase the effects of Dilantin include coumarin-type anticoagulants, disulfiram, phenylbutazone, isoniazid, chloramphenicol, cimetidine, sulfa drugs, and dexamethasone.
- Drugs that decrease the effects of Dilantin include barbiturates, carbamazepine, folic acid supplements, calcium supplements, central nervous system depressants, antacids, oxacillin, and some cancer drugs.
- Dilanin decreases the effects of the following drugs: dicumarol, disopyramide, quinidine, corticosteroid drugs, digitoxin, and furosemide.

- Dilantin increases the effects of warfarin.

Other:
- Do not discontinue medication or change dosage without talking with your doctor.
- To prevent overgrowth of gum tissue, maintain good oral hygiene, including flossing and gum massage.
- If this drug causes drowsiness, be certain that you are careful when engaging in activities that require alertness.
- There are other drugs that contain phenytoin, but they are not equivalent to Dilantin. Do not switch brands or request a generic drug without talking to your doctor.
- Phenobarbital is also prescribed for epilepsy.
- You should carry an identification card stating that you have epilepsy and are taking Dilantin.
- If you are diabetic, monitor urine sugar regularly and send any abnormal results to your doctor.

Medical Tests:

- Your doctor may want to perform periodic lab tests, including liver function, blood counts, and urinalysis, to monitor your progress while taking this drug.
- Dilantin may affect the results of blood and urine tests.
- Usage is monitored by measuring blood levels.
- Any drug may affect the results and accuracy of a medical test. If a doctor recommends a medical or laboratory test for any condition, inform the doctor that you are taking this drug.

DIMETAPP

Ingredient(s): phenylpropanolamine, phenylephrine hydrochloride, brompheniramine

Equivalent Product(s): Bromalix, Bromatapp, Bromophen, Bromphen Compound, Cordamine-PA, Dimalix, Dimaphen, E-Tapp, Histatapp, Midatap, Normatane, Purebrom, S-T Decongest SF and DF, Tagatap, Tamine, Trancaps Capsules, Tri-Phen, Veltap

Used for: relief of allergy symptoms

Dosage Form and Strength: elixir—5 mg phenylpropanolamine, 5 mg phenylephrine hydrochloride, 4 mg brompheniramine per 5 ml; tablets—15 mg phenylpropanolamine, 15 mg phenylephrine hydrochloride, 12 mg brompheniramine

Storage: Store at room temperature.

Before Using This Drug, Tell Your Doctor: if you have a history of asthma, high blood pressure, heart disease, circulatory disease, diabetes, ulcers, thyroid problems, glaucoma, seizures, enlarged prostate, or urinary or intestinal tract obstruction. Also, tell your doctor about any drug, prescription or nonprescription, you are using and about any allergies you have or any family history of allergies.

This Drug Should Not Be Used If: you are allergic to its ingredients; have high blood pressure, a heart condition, glaucoma, or an obstructed bladder; or are taking certain antidepressants (MAO inhibitors). This drug should not be used to treat asthma.

How to Use: Take the medication with a glass of water or with food or milk. Measure the liquid in a medical teaspoon. Swallow the tablets whole; do not crush or chew them.

Time Required for Drug to Take Effect: approximately 30 minutes to one hour

Missing a Dose: Take the missed dose as soon as you remember. However, if it is almost time for the next dose, do not take the missed dose; return to the regular schedule. Do not double the next dose.

Symptoms of Overdose: excitement, clumsiness, muscle spasms, hallucinations, convulsions, dilated pupils, flushed face, fever, shallow breathing, weak and rapid pulse, headache, sweating, nausea, vomiting

Side Effects:

Minor and expected:
- drowsiness, thickening of lung and respiratory secretions, nausea, vomiting, diarrhea, constipation, dizziness, nervousness, restless sleeping, headache, dry mouth, loss of appetite

Serious adverse reactions (CALL YOUR DOCTOR):
- vision disturbances, skin rash, hives, tight chest, unusual bleeding or bruising, fast or pounding heartbeat, chest pain, unexplained sore throat and fever, clumsiness, unusual weakness, ringing in the ears, difficult or painful urination

Effects of Long-Term Use: This type of medication should not be used for a prolonged period of time. If it is used too long, it may produce involuntary movements of lips, tongue, and jaw; possible reduction in the ability of the bone marrow, the soft connective tissue inside the bones, to do its job of manufacturing blood cells; and worsening of congestion rather than relief.

Habit-Forming Possibility: none, unless it is used so frequently or for so long that the body becomes dependent on the drug to perform the functions the body would normally do

Precautions and Suggestions:

Foods and beverages:
- No food restrictions.
- Avoid alcohol.

Other medicines, prescription and nonprescription:
- This drug may interact with other antihistamines, anticoagulants, amphetamines, antidepressants (especially MAO inhibitors), medications for cough and colds, asthma and breathing medicines, narcotics, painkillers, seizure medicine, sedatives, tranquilizers, sleeping medications, debrisoquin, guanethidine, levodopa, ammonium chloride, and beta blockers.

Other:
- If this drug causes you to become drowsy, do not engage in activities that require alertness, such as driving a car or operating potentially dangerous machinery.
- Call your doctor if this drug causes excited or overstimulated behavior.

Medical Tests:
- Your doctor may want to take blood cell counts while this medication is being used.
- Any drug may affect the results and accuracy of a medical test. If a doctor recommends a medical or laboratory test for any condition, inform the doctor that you are taking this drug.
- *Note:* This drug recently became available over the counter. It is listed here because it is important that all of the information about it be known since it contains multiple ingredients.

DONNATAL

Ingredient(s): atropine sulfate, scopolamine hydrobromide, hyoscyamine hydrobromide, phenobarbital

Equivalent Product(s): Barophen, Bay-Ase, belladonna alkaloids with phenobarbital, Bellalphen, Bellastal, Donnamor, Donna-Sed, Hyosophen, Malatal, Neoquess, Palbar, Pylora, Relaxadon, Seds, Spasaid, Spaslin, Spasmolin, Spasmophen, Susano, Vanatal

Used for: intestinal disorders such as irritable bowel, spastic colon, various types of colitis, and duodenal ulcer

Dosage Form and Strength: tablets—0.0194 mg atropine sulfate, 0.0065 mg scopolamine hydrobromide, 0.1037 mg hyoscyamine hydrobromide, 16.2 mg phenobarbital; 0.0194 mg atropine sulfate, 0.0065 mg scopolamine hydrobromide, 0.1037 mg hyoscyamine hydrobromide, 32.4 mg phenobarbital; 0.0582 mg atropine sulfate, 0.0195 mg scopolamine hydrobromide, 0.3111 mg hyoscyamine hydrobromide, 48.6 mg phenobarbital (Extentabs); elixir—0.0194 mg atropine sulfate, 0.0065 scopolamine hydrobromide, 0.1037 mg hyoscyamine hydrobromide, 16 mg phenobarbital per 5 ml

Storage: Store in a tightly closed container away from light.

Before Using This Drug, Tell Your Doctor: if you have glaucoma, other eye disorders, rapid heartbeat, heart disease, high blood pressure, kidney or liver disease, obstruction in gastrointestinal or urinary tract, lack of intestinal muscle tone, ulcerative colitis, myasthenia gravis, lung disease, hiatal hernia, enlarged prostate, overactive thyroid gland, diabetes, epilepsy, anemia, disorders of adrenal glands, porphyria, or asthma. Tell your doctor about any drugs, prescription or nonprescription, you are taking and about any allergies you have or any family history of allergies.

This Drug Should Not Be Used If: you are allergic to any of its ingredients or if you have glaucoma, adhesions between iris and lens of eye, rapid heartbeat, certain heart conditions, kidney or liver disease, porphyria, obstruction in gastrointestinal or urinary tract, lack of intestinal muscle tone, complications of ulcerative colitis, myasthenia gravis, or chronic lung disease.

How to Use: Take Donnatal 30 minutes before a meal. Do not crush the Extentabs; take them whole. Antacids interfere with the absorption of Donnatal; do not use an antacid within an hour of taking this medication.

Time Required for Drug to Take Effect: Effects begin in one to two hours.

Missing a Dose: Omit the missed dose and maintain your regular schedule. At the next dose time, do not take the missed dose and do not double the next dose.

Symptoms of Overdose: extreme dryness of mouth, difficulty in swallowing, vomiting, nausea, abdominal bloating, abdominal pain, muscle weakness, confusion, extreme drowsiness, delirium, fever, headache, restlessness, excited state, lethargy, depression, tremor, hallucinations, loss of consciousness, unusual changes in behavior, heartbeat irregularities, rapid pulse and breathing, pounding heartbeat, rise in blood pressure, difficult urination, blurred vision, dilated pupils, increase in body temperature, flushed and hot skin, rash, breathing difficulty

Side Effects:

Minor and expected:
- dry mouth and throat, change in taste perception, heartburn, bloated feeling, nasal congestion, drowsiness, decrease in sweating, constipation, slightly blurred vision, increased sensitivity to light, hesitancy in urination

Serious adverse reactions (CALL YOUR DOCTOR):
- nausea, vomiting, changes in speech, urine retention, difficult urination, impotence, dilated pupils, eye pain, changes in heartbeat, headaches, nervousness, weakness, dizziness, insomnia, restlessness, tremor, unexplained fever, delirium, rash, hives, flushed and dry skin, confusion, changes in behavior, difficult breathing, yellowish discoloration of skin and whites of eyes

Effects of Long-Term Use: chronic constipation

Habit-Forming Possibility: This drug should be used with care because one of its ingredients, phenobarbital, can lead to physical and psychological dependence.

Precautions and Suggestions:

Foods and beverages:
- No food restrictions, although your doctor may recommend a special diet for your condition.
- Ask your doctor if you can use alcohol.

Other medicines, prescription and nonprescription:
- Donnatal can interact with some anesthetics; tell your doctor or dentist that you are taking this drug before any procedure that requires an anesthetic.
- Donnatal may interact with medicines for colds, cough, or allergies.

- Other drugs similar to Donnatal may increase the side effects of Donnatal. These drugs include antihistamines, antipsychotics, drugs for Parkinson's disease, alphaprodine, buclizine, meperidine, orphenadrine, benzodiazepines, certain antidepressants, methylphenidate, nitrates, nitrites, alkalinizing agents, primidone, thioxanthenes, procainamide, quinidine, monoamine oxidase inhibitors.
- Donnatal may also interact with corticosteroids, haloperidol, cholinesterase inhibitors, guanethidine, histamine, reserpine, digitalis, digoxin, cholinergics, diphenhydramine, drugs for lung and respiratory conditions, anticonvulsants, some antibiotics, anticoagulants, digitoxin, furosemide, antidiabetic drugs, isoniazid, and pilocarpine drops for glaucoma.

Other:

- If this drug causes drowsiness or blurred vision, do not engage in activities that require alertness, such as driving a car or operating potentially dangerous equipment.
- If this drug causes a decrease in sweating, avoid strenuous activity in hot weather, saunas, and hot baths in order to prevent heatstroke.

Medical Tests:

- Your doctor may want to measure your eye pressure at periodic intervals.
- Donnatal also may interfere with the results of liver function tests, thyroid function tests, and some blood and urine tests.
- Any drug may affect the results and accuracy of a medical test. If a doctor recommends a medical or laboratory test for any condition, inform the doctor that you are taking this drug.

DYAZIDE

Ingredient(s): triamterene and hydrochlorothiazide

Equivalent Product(s): none

Used for: treatment of high blood pressure and removal of excessive fluid from the body. Generally, a drug that lowers the body's fluid level also lowers the potassium level. Dyazide, however, is a potassium-sparing drug, which means that it does not remove potassium (important for maintaining chemical balance) from the body as it removes the fluid.

Dosage Form and Strength: capsules—50 mg triamterene and 25 mg hydrochlorothiazide

Storage: Store in a dry, tightly sealed, light-resistant container.

Before Using This Drug, Tell Your Doctor: about any allergic reactions—especially asthmatic—that you've had to this drug and/or its ingredients or to any sulfa drugs. Also tell your doctor if you have any other allergies and/or a history of asthma, diabetes, gout, heart disease, liver or kidney disease, kidney stones, problems with urinating, anemia, blood diseases, systemic lupus erythematosus, pancreas disorders, and high levels of calcium or potassium in your body. Be certain to tell your doctor about any medicines, prescription or nonprescription, that you are taking.

This Drug Should Not Be Used If: you have severe or progressive liver or kidney disease, difficulty in urinating, or high blood levels of potassium. Also, if you are allergic to the ingredients of Dyazide or to sulfa drugs, you should not take this medicine. You should not use Dyazide if you are taking other potassium-sparing drugs, such as spironolactone.

How to Use: Take this drug with food or milk and exactly as directed.

Time Required for Drug to Take Effect: Increased urination begins in one hour, peaks in two to three hours, and subsides in seven to nine hours.

Missing a Dose: Take the missed dose as soon as you remember and continue with your usual schedule. However, if it is nearly time for the next dose, skip the missed dose and remain on the usual schedule. Do not double the dose or take extra.

Symptoms of Overdose: excessive urination, fatigue, thirst, nausea, vomiting, weakness, fever, and flushed face

Side Effects:

Minor and expected:
- fatigue, constipation, diarrhea, drowsiness, light-headedness, loss of appetite, upset stomach, and increased sensitivity to the sun. Dyazide may turn your urine blue in color; this is a harmless reaction.

Serious adverse reactions (CALL YOUR DOCTOR):

- dizziness; dry mouth; increased thirst; nausea; vomiting; fever and sore throat; flushed face; muscle cramps; numbness or tingling in hands, feet, or lips; mood changes; continuing weakness or fatigue; fever; mouth sores, rash, or hives; irregular or weak pulse; unusual bleeding or bruising; yellowish tinge to skin or whites of eyes.

Effects of Long-Term Use: accumulation of potassium in the body, causing higher than normal blood levels of potassium. This can affect the body's proper regulation of heart rhythm.

Habit-Forming Possibility: none

Precautions and Suggestions:

Foods and beverages:

- Your doctor may give you instructions about the use of potassium-rich foods and beverages as well as about the amount of salt you can eat. Ask your doctor about the use of salt substitutes, many of which contain potassium.
- Use alcohol with caution; alcohol can increase the blood pressure–lowering action of this drug, leading to abnormally low blood pressure.

Other medicines, prescription and nonprescription:

- Because this drug does not cause the loss of potassium as other fluid-lowering drugs do, you should not take any potassium supplements while using Dyazide unless instructed to do so by your doctor. Dyazide also may interact with calcium salts and vitamin D supplements.
- This drug interacts with other high blood pressure drugs (especially spironolactone, captopril, and diazoxide), fenfluramine, quinidine, furosemide, sulfonamides, some muscle relaxants, curare, digitalis, lithium carbonate, cortisone and other steroids, oral antidiabetic drugs and insulin, gout drugs (Benemid, Zyloprim), tricyclic antidepressants (Elavil, Sinequan), monoamine oxidase (MAO) inhibitors, barbiturates, pain relievers (both narcotic and nonnarcotic), indomethacin and other nonsteroid anti-inflammatory drugs, cholestyramine (Cuemid, Questran, colestipol), quinidine, anticoagulants (Coumadin), sulfa drugs, and beta blockers (Inderal and Lopressor). Also, do not take any nonprescription medicines for weight control or cough, cold, or sinus problems without consulting your doctor.

Other:

- If this drug makes you dizzy or drowsy, do not drive a car, operate machinery, or participate in any activity that requires alertness.
- Because this drug may increase sensitivity to sunlight, use caution in the sun until your sensitivity has been determined.
- Before you have any kind of surgery or dental treatment, tell your doctor or dentist that you are taking Dyazide.
- Avoid strenuous activity that could increase perspiration and thus cause additional loss of fluid and salt from the body.
- If you develop an illness that causes diarrhea or vomiting, call your doctor. Both diarrhea and vomiting can upset the fluid balance of the body.

Medical Tests:

- Your doctor may recommend periodic tests to monitor the effects of this drug in the body, including complete blood counts; measurements of blood levels of potassium, sodium, chloride, sugar, and uric acid; and liver, kidney, and thyroid function tests. Dyazide can interfere with the results of thyroid function tests.
- Any drug may affect the results and accuracy of a medical test. If a doctor recommends a medical or laboratory test for any condition, inform the doctor that you are taking Dyazide.

ERYTHROMYCIN (GENERIC)

Ingredient(s): erythromycin

Equivalent Product(s): Bristamycin, E.E.S., E-Mycin, Eramycin, Eryc, Erypar, EryPed, Ery-Tab, Erythrocin, Ethril, Ilosone, Pediamycin, Pfizer-E, SK-Erythromycin, Wyamycin

Used for: a wide variety of bacterial infections

Dosage Form and Strength: tablets (includes chewable and enteric or film-coated), capsules, drops, and oral suspension—various strengths

Storage: Store liquid forms of this drug in the refrigerator. Store other forms in tightly closed containers at room temperature.

Before Using This Drug, Tell Your Doctor: if you have a history of bronchial asthma, kidney disease, sensitivity to aspirin, or liver disease. Also tell your doctor about any drugs, prescription or nonprescription, that you are using (especially bronchodilators, anticonvulsants, and other antibiotics) and about any known allergies or any family history of allergies.

This Drug Should Not Be Used If: you are allergic to erythromycin or have liver disease.

How to Use: This drug preferably should be taken on an empty stomach, one hour before or two hours after a meal. However, if stomach upset occurs, you can take this drug with food. Some types of erythromycin can be taken without regard to food or meals. Ask your doctor which type is being prescribed for you. If you are using the oral suspension, shake the bottle well and measure the dose with a medical teaspoon. If you are giving drops to an elderly person, measure the medicine in a marked dropper and release the liquid into the inside of the person's cheek. Take each dose with at least one-half to one full glass of water. Take the medication at evenly spaced intervals, preferably around the clock. Take the full amount of medication until it is gone, even if you seem and feel well.

Time Required for Drug to Take Effect: varies, depending on the illness being treated

Missing a Dose: Take the missed dose immediately. If you do not remember to take the missed dose until almost time for the next dose, space that next dose about midway through the normal interval between doses. For example, if you are to take a dose at 8:00 A.M., noon, 4:00 P.M., and 8:00 P.M., and you remember at 7:00 P.M. that you forgot the 4:00 P.M. dose, take the missed dose at 7:00, but wait until 10:00 P.M. to take the 8:00 P.M. dose. Then return to your normal schedule. Do not skip a dose.

Symptoms of Overdose: severe nausea, vomiting, abdominal discomfort, diarrhea

Side Effects:

Minor and expected:
- nausea, vomiting, diarrhea, stomach cramps

Serious adverse reactions (CALL YOUR DOCTOR):
- severe abdominal pain, yellow discoloration of skin or whites of eyes, dark urine, pale-colored stools, unusual fatigue, hearing loss, rash, itching, superinfection, mood changes, itching in genital or anal area

Effects of Long-Term Use: superinfection—a second infection in addition to the infection being treated. The superinfection is caused by bacteria and other organisms that are not susceptible to or affected by the drug being used to treat the original infection. Thus, these organisms, which normally are too few in number to cause problems, grow unchecked and cause a second infection that may require treatment with a different drug.

Habit-Forming Possibility: none

Precautions and Suggestions:

Foods and beverages:
- No restrictions.

Other medicines, prescription and nonprescription:
- Erythromycin may affect the effects of theophylline or carbamazepine in the body. Be sure to tell your doctor if you are taking theophylline for asthma or breathing problems or carbamazepine for epilepsy.
- This drug may interact with digoxin and oral anticoagulants.
- Some of the forms of erythromycin contain a dye called *tartrazine*, which may cause allergic-type reactions (including bronchial asthma) in some people, especially those sensitive to aspirin.

Other:
- If mild diarrhea is a side effect, ask your doctor if you can eat yogurt. The beneficial bacteria in yogurt replace the intestine's natural beneficial bacteria that have been reduced or eliminated by erythromycin.
- Do not use the medication beyond the expiration date on the container.
- If you have any doubts about how you are reacting to the medication, call your doctor.

Medical Tests:

- Erythromycin interferes with urine laboratory tests.
- Any drug may affect the results and accuracy of a medical test. If a doctor recommends a medical or laboratory test for any condition, inform the doctor that you are taking this drug.

FELDENE

Ingredient(s): piroxicam

Equivalent Product(s): none

Used for: relief of symptoms of arthritis

Dosage Form and Strength: capsules—10 mg, 20 mg

Storage: Store in a tightly closed container.

Before Using This Drug, Tell Your Doctor: if you have a history of stomach problems, ulcers, ulcerative colitis, kidney disease, urination problems, liver disease, heart disease, bleeding or clotting problems, circulatory problems, anemia, high blood pressure, Parkinson's disease, epilepsy, or vision disorders. Tell your doctor about any drugs, prescription or nonprescription, you are taking, especially anticoagulant drugs. Tell your doctor about any allergies you have, particularly to aspirin or similar drugs, and about any family history of allergies.

This Drug Should Not Be Used If: you are allergic to its ingredient, to any other similar nonsteroid anti-inflammatory drugs, or to aspirin and salicylates.

How to Use: Try taking the drug on an empty stomach. However, if stomach upset occurs, take the medication with food. Also, ask your doctor if you can take the drug with an antacid if stomach upset is a problem. Do not take aspirin at the same time you are using Feldene.

Time Required for Drug to Take Effect: seven to 12 days

Missing a Dose: Take the missed dose as soon as you remember, unless it is almost time for the next dose. In that case, omit the missed dose and maintain your regular dosing schedule. Do not double the next dose.

Symptoms of Overdose: To date, there is no record of overdose cases, so symptoms are not known.

Side Effects:

Minor and expected:
- upset somach, heartburn, nausea, vomiting, indigestion, constipation, diarrhea, dry mouth, drowsiness, headache, blurred vision, bloated feeling, gas, runny nose, loss of appetite, peculiar taste in mouth

Serious adverse reactions (CALL YOUR DOCTOR):
- severe abdominal pain, black tarry or bloody stool, rectal bleeding, yellowish discoloration of skin and whites of eyes, mouth sores, sleep disorders, nervousness, feeling of numbness or tingling, tremor, convulsions, muscle weakness or pain, fatigue, confusion, depression, emotional disturbances, urination or kidney problems, unusual bleeding or bruising, eye disorders, ringing in the ears, impaired hearing, ear pain, breathing difficulty, rash, hives, itching, hair loss, weight gain, retention of fluid, persistent headache, unexplained sore throat and fever, heartbeat irregularities, chest pain, changes in blood pressure

Effects of Long-Term Use: possible development of anemia

Habit-Forming Possibility: none

Precautions and Suggestions:

Foods and beverages:
- No food restrictions.
- Ask your doctor if you can drink alcoholic beverages.

Other medicines, prescription and nonprescription:
- Feldene may interact with oral antidiabetic drugs, anticonvulsants, sulfa drugs, probenecid, steroids, and other arthritis medications.
- If you are taking coumarin-type anticoagulants, Feldene can affect blood clotting.
- Aspirin decreases the effectiveness of Feldene; therefore, aspirin should not be taken at the same time.

Other:
- If this drug makes you dizzy or drowsy or causes blurred vision, avoid activities that require alertness, such as driving a car or operating potentially dangerous machinery.
- Because of its anti-inflammatory and fever-reducing qualities, this drug may mask the symptoms of an infection. If you suspect an infection is developing, call your doctor.
- Do not stop taking this drug suddenly or increase the dosage without consulting your doctor.

Medical Tests:
- Your doctor may want to perform blood tests as well as liver and kidney function tests to monitor your progress on this drug.
- If you have impaired hearing or vision, you will probably be told to have regular vision and hearing tests.
- Any drug may affect the results and accuracy of a medical test. If a doctor recommends a medical or laboratory test for any condition, inform the doctor that you are taking this drug.

FIORINAL

Ingredient(s): butalbital, aspirin, caffeine

Equivalent Product(s): Buff-A-Comp, butalbital with aspirin and caffeine (generic), Butal Compound, Isollyl (Improved), Lanorinal, Marnal, Protension, Tenstan

Used for: relief of anxiety and tension as well as insomnia

Dosage Form and Strength: capsules and tablets—50 mg, butalbital, 325 mg aspirin, 40 mg caffeine

Storage: Store in a tightly closed container.

Before Using This Drug, Tell Your Doctor: if you have liver or kidney disease, porphyria, respiratory or lung problems, epilepsy, thyroid disorders, diabetes, anemia, heart disease, bleeding or clotting disorders, peptic ulcer, gout, urination difficulties, or a history of drug dependence. Tell your doctor about any drugs, prescription or nonprescription, you are taking and about any allergies you have or any family history of allergies.

This Drug Should Not Be Used If: you have an allergy to any of its ingredients or to any similar drugs (such as barbiturates). This drug should not be used by those with porphyria, liver disease, kidney disease, severe respiratory disease, active peptic ulcer, bleeding disorders (such as hemophilia), or a history of drug dependence. This drug should not be taken by anyone already taking anticoagulants.

How to Use: Take this drug with a glass of water or with food to prevent stomach upset.

Time Required for Drug to Take Effect: begins to take effect in 15 to 30 minutes, reaches its effectiveness in one hour, and begins to subside in two to six hours

Missing a Dose: Take the missed dose as soon as you remember within an hour of the regular dosage time. If more than an hour has passed, do not take the missed dose but maintain your regular dosing schedule. Do not double the next dose.

Symptoms of Overdose: confusion, slurred speech, drowsiness, clumsiness, reduced urine volume, staggering walk, slow and shallow breathing, weak and rapid pulse, cold and sweaty skin, ringing in ears, deep sleep, lowered body temperature, eventually loss of consciousness

Side Effects:

Minor and expected:
- drowsiness, sleepiness, a hangover feeling, dizziness, nausea, vomiting, diarrhea, constipation, headache, muscle pain, joint ache

Serious adverse reactions (CALL YOUR DOCTOR):
- sore throat, fever, mouth sores, easy bruising, nosebleed, purplish spots on skin, skin rash, hives, swelling around the face, difficult breathing, wheezing, tightness in the chest, slow heartbeat, fatigue,

extreme sleepiness during the day, yellowish discoloration of the skin and whites of eyes, confusion, headache, unsteadiness, unusual nervousness or excitement, nightmares, hallucinations, delirium, impaired vision, sleeplessness, anxiety, depression

Effects of Long-Term Use: anemia, dependence, possible kidney damage and aggravation of stomach ulcer, prolongation of bleeding time

Habit-Forming Possibility: This drug can lead to both physical and psychological dependence. This drug has potential for abuse since tolerance to it can develop easily.

Precautions and Suggestions:

Foods and beverages:
- No food restrictions, but remember that coffee, tea, colas, and chocolate contain caffeine, one of the ingredients in this drug.
- Avoid alcoholic beverages.

Other medicines, prescription and nonprescription:
- This drug may interact with anticonvulsants, central nervous system depressants (sedatives, other sleeping aids, antihistamines, tranquilizers, phenothiazines, alchohol), antidepressants, antibiotics (tetracycline, doxycycline, chloramphenicol), anticoagulants, the antifungal griseofulvin, sulfa drugs, steroid drugs, thyroid drugs, amphetamines, monoamine oxidase inhibitors, digitoxin, quinidine, methotrexate, furosemide, antidiabetic drugs, isoniazid, theophylline, and aminophylline.

Other:
- If this drug causes you to become drowsy, do not engage in activities that require alertness.
- In older persons, this drug may cause a reduction in the body temperature (hypothermia). During cold weather, keep dosage to a minimum and dress warmly.
- Do not change the prescribed dosage without consulting a doctor.
- Do not stop taking this drug abruptly; if you have been taking this drug for an extended period of time, you must stop using the drug gradually.

Medical Tests:

- Your doctor may want to conduct tests to monitor the therapy.
- This drug may affect the results of some blood and urine tests.
- Any drug may affect the results and accuracy of a medical test. If a doctor recommends a medical or laboratory test for any condition, inform the doctor that you are taking this drug.

GANTRISIN

Ingredient(s): sulfisoxazole

Equivalent Product(s): SK-Soxazole, sulfisoxazole (generic), Sulfizin

Used for: treatment of a variety of bacterial infections, especially in the urinary tract

Dosage Form and Strength: tablets—500 mg; syrup—500 mg per 5 ml teaspoon; pediatric suspension—500 mg per 5 ml teaspoon

Storage: Store in a tightly closed container at room temperature.

Before Using This Drug, Tell Your Doctor: if you have any kidney or liver disorders; an obstruction in the urinary or intestinal tract; strep throat; a history of allergies, anemia, or bronchial asthma; or porphyria; G6PD deficiency. Also, tell your doctor about any drugs, prescription or nonprescription, that you are using and about any allergies you have or any family history of allergies.

This Drug Should Not Be Used If: you are allergic to its ingredient or to any sulfa drugs or thiazide diuretics. This drug should not be used if you have a urinary or intestinal obstruction or if you have strep throat or porphyria.

How to Use: This drug should be taken on an empty stomach at least one hour before or two hours after meals with a full glass of water. However, if stomach upset occurs, you can take this drug with food. Drink as much water as possible during the day—preferably eight glasses. If you are using the liquid versions of this drug, shake the bottle thoroughly and measure with a medical teaspoon. Give the medicine at evenly spaced intervals around the clock. Give the full amount of medication until it is gone, even if you seem and feel well.

Time Required for Drug to Take Effect: varies, depending on the illness being treated; usually two to five days

Missing a Dose: Take the missed dose as soon as you remember, unless it is almost time for the next dose. In that case if you are taking three or more doses a day, space the missed dose and the next dose two to four hours apart. Then return to your regular dosing schedule.

Symptoms of Overdose: severe nausea, vomiting, dizziness, headache, drowsiness, yellowing of skin and whites of eyes, fever, and loss of consciousness

Side Effects:

Minor and expected:
- loss of appetite, nausea, vomiting, depression, headache, dizziness, sleeplessness, and sensitivity to sunlight. This drug will also cause a brown discoloration of the urine, which is harmless.

Serious adverse reactions (CALL YOUR DOCTOR):
- unexplained sore throat or fever, paleness, purplish or yellowish discoloration of the skin, rash, itching (especially in genital and anal areas), abdominal pains, bloody diarrhea, difficulty in urination, reduced amount of urine, unusual bleeding or bruising, pain in muscles and joints, breathing or swallowing difficulties, hearing loss, ringing in the ears, loss of coordination, convulsions, hair loss, blood in urine, chills, swelling of the face or neck, or mouth sores

Effects of Long-Term Use: superinfection—a second infection in addition to the infection being treated. The superinfection is caused by bacteria and other organisms that are not susceptible to or affected by the drug being used to treat the original infection. Thus, these organisms, which normally are too few in number to cause problems, grow unchecked and cause a second infection that may require treatment with a different drug. Also possible enlargement of the thyroid gland with or without impaired functioning of the gland

Habit-Forming Possibility: none

Precautions and Suggestions:

Foods and beverages:
- No food restrictions.
- Ask your doctor about drinking alcoholic beverages while taking this drug.

Other medicines, prescription and nonprescription:
- Gantrisin may interact with aspirin-type drugs (salicylates), the anticonvulsant phenytoin, methenamines, antibiotics, local anesthetics, and para-aminobenzoic acid (PABA) that is found in some sunscreens.
- It also interacts with some oral diabetes drugs (tolbutamide, chlorpropamide), warfarin, methotrexate, phenylbutazone, probenecid, digoxin, and ferrous sulfate and interferes with folic acid absorption.

Other:
- If this drug causes you to become increasingly sensitive to the sun, be certain that you are protected from exposure to the sun, but do not use a sunscreen with PABA in it.

- If this drug causes drowsiness or dizziness, do not engage in activity requiring alertness.

Medical Tests:

- Your doctor may want to perform blood and urine tests to monitor your progress while taking this drug.
- Gantrisin can interfere with the results of urine tests for glucose (sugar) and protein.
- Any drug may affect the results and accuracy of a medical test. If a doctor recommends a medical or laboratory test for any condition, inform the doctor that you are taking this drug.

HYDROCHLOROTHIAZIDE (GENERIC)

Ingredient(s): hydrochlorothiazide

Equivalent Product(s): Aquazide, Chlozide, Diaqua, Diu-Scrip, Esidrix, Hydro-Chlor, HydroDiuril, Hydromal, Hydro-T, Hydro-Z-50, Mictrin, Oretic, SK-Hydrochlorothiazide, Thiuretic, Zide

Used for: treatment of high blood pressure. It is also used to eliminate fluid retention caused by disorders such as heart failure, cirrhosis of the liver, and kidney disease, as well as the long-term use of some drugs.

Dosage Form and Strength: tablets—25 mg, 50 mg, 100 mg,

Storage: Store in a dry, tightly closed container.

Before Using This Drug, Tell Your Doctor: if you have kidney or liver disease, bronchial asthma, lupus erythematosus, gout, or diabetes. Tell your doctor about any drugs, prescription or nonprescription, you are taking, especially cortisone, gout medicines, digitalis, oral antidiabetes drugs, or insulin. Tell your doctor about any allergies you have, especially to sulfa drugs, and about any family history of allergies.

This Drug Should Not Be Used If: you have a history of kidney disease or are allergic to its ingredient or to sulfa drugs.

How to Use: Take with food or milk to prevent stomach upset.

Time Required for Drug to Take Effect: Urine output will increase in about two hours, reach a peak in four to six hours, and return to normal in about eight to 12 hours. Your doctor will probably want you to take the drug for two to three weeks and then test to see if this drug is effective for your condition.

Missing a Dose: Take the missed dose as soon as you remember, unless it is almost time for the next dose. In that case, omit the missed dose and simply maintain your regular dosing schedule. Do not double the next dose.

Symptoms of Overdose: confusion, dizziness, muscle weakness, upset stomach, breathing difficulty, lethargy, loss of consciousness, seizures

Side Effects:

Minor and expected:
- increased frequency of urination, diarrhea, loss of appetite, mild upset stomach, abdominal cramps, constipation, sensitivity to sunlight, drowsiness, headache

Serious adverse reactions (CALL YOUR DOCTOR):
- muscle weakness or cramps, light-headedness, nausea, dizziness, dizziness upon standing up, confusion, vomiting, yellowish discoloration of skin and whites of eyes, impotence, decreased interest in sex, restlessness, insomnia, fainting, unexplained fever or sore throat, irregular heartbeat, chest pain, purplish discoloration of skin, rash, hives, itching, breathing problems, temporary blurred vision, chills, flushing, weight loss, weight gain, dry mouth, excessive thirst

Effects of Long-Term Use: possible imbalance of water, salt, and potassium in body tissues; development of diabetes in susceptible people

Habit-Forming Possibility: none

Precautions and Suggestions:

Foods and beverages:
- Your doctor may recommend a low-salt, high-potassium diet. This drug helps remove water from your body and at the same time may remove potassium.Therefore, ask your doctor about foods that are rich in potassium.
- Avoid licorice while using this drug.
- Ask your doctor if you can drink alcoholic beverages.

Other medicines, prescription and nonprescription:
- Hydrochlorothiazide may increase the effects of other drugs for high blood pressure, phenothiazines, narcotics, decongestants, or bronchodilators.
- This drug may decrease the effects of oral antidiabetics and insulin, as well as gout medicines.
- The effects of this drug may be decreased by cholestyramine and colestipol.
- The effects of this drug may be increased by barbiturates, monoamine oxidase inhibitors, and narcotic and nonnarcotic pain relievers.
- Hydrochlorothiazide may also interact with indomethacin, steroids, digitalis, norepinephrine, some antidepressants, calcium salts, vitamin D, diazoxide, furosemide, other diuretics, sulfa drugs, fenfluramine, quinidine, and lithium.

Other:
- If this drug makes you dizzy or drowsy, do not engage in activities that require alertness, such as driving a car or operating potentially dangerous machinery.
- Avoid strenuous activity or becoming overheated in hot weather; this may cause extra loss of water from your body because of excessive perspiration.
- If you have an illness that causes diarrhea or vomiting, call your doctor.
- If you develop a sensitivity to sunlight, protect yourself with clothing and a sunscreen before exposure to sunlight.
- Ask your doctor if you can take this drug early in the day to avoid getting up at night to urinate.
- Before any surgery, tell your doctor, surgeon, or dentist that you are taking this drug.

Medical Tests:

- Your doctor may want to perform periodic laboratory tests to monitor your progress on this drug, especially if you are diabetic or have gout. He or she will also want to monitor your water-salt-potassium levels during this treatment.
- Hydrochlorothiazide may affect the results of some blood and urine tests, including tests for thyroid and parathyroid function.
- Any drug may affect the results and accuracy of a medical test. If a doctor recommends a medical or laboratory test for any condition, inform the doctor that you are taking this drug.

HYGROTON

Ingredient(s): chlorthalidone

Equivalent Product(s): chlorthalidone (generic), Hylidone, Thalitone

Used for: treatment of high blood pressure. It is also used to eliminate fluid retention caused by disorders such as heart failure, cirrhosis of the liver, and kidney disease, as well as the long-term use of some drugs.

Dosage Form and Strength: tablets—25 mg, 50 mg, 100 mg

Storage: Store in a dry, tightly closed container.

Before Using This Drug, Tell Your Doctor: if you have kidney or liver disease, bronchial asthma, lupus erythematosus, gout, or diabetes. Tell your doctor about any drugs, prescription or nonprescription, you are taking, especially cortisone, gout medicines, digitalis, oral antidiabetic medications, or insulin. Tell your doctor about any allergies you have, especially to sulfa drugs, and about any family history of allergies.

This Drug Should Not Be Used If: you have a history of kidney disease or are allergic to its ingredient or to sulfa drugs.

How to Use: Take with food or milk to prevent stomach upset.

Time Required for Drug to Take Effect: Urine output will increase in about two hours, reach a peak in six to 18 hours, and return to normal in 48 to 72 hours. Your doctor will probably want you to take the drug for two to three weeks and then test to see if this drug is effective for your condition.

Missing a Dose: Take the missed dose as soon as you remember, unless it is almost time for the next dose. In that case, omit the missed dose and simply maintain your regular dosing schedule. Do not double the next dose.

Symptoms of Overdose: confusion, dizziness, muscle weakness, upset stomach, breathing difficulty, lethargy, loss of consciousness, seizures

Side Effects:

Minor and expected:
- increased frequency of urination, diarrhea, loss of appetite, mild upset stomach, abdominal cramps, constipation, sensitivity to sunlight, drowsiness, headache

Serious adverse reactions (CALL YOUR DOCTOR):
- muscle weakness or cramps, light-headedness, nausea, dizziness, dizziness upon standing up, confusion, vomiting, yellowish discoloration of skin and whites of eyes, impotence, decreased interest in sex, restlessness, insomnia, fainting, unexplained sore throat and fever, irregular heartbeat, chest pain, purplish discoloration of skin, rash, hives, itching, breathing problems, temporarily blurred vision, chills, flushing, weight loss or gain, dry mouth, excessive thirst

Effects of Long-Term Use: possible imbalance of water, salt, and potassium in body tissues; development of diabetes in susceptible people

Habit-Forming Possibility: none

Precautions and Suggestions:

Foods and beverages:
- Your doctor may recommend a low-salt, high-potassium diet. This drug helps remove water from your body and at the same time may remove potassium. Therefore, ask your doctor about foods that are rich in potassium.
- Avoid licorice while taking this drug.
- Ask your doctor if you can drink alcoholic beverages.

Other medicines, prescription and nonprescription:
- Hygroton may increase the effects of other drugs for high blood pressure, phenothiazines, narcotics, decongestants, or bronchodilators.
- This drug may decrease the effects of oral antidiabetics and insulin as well as gout medications.
- The effects of this drug may be decreased by cholestyramine and colestipol.
- The effects of this drug may be increased by barbiturates, monoamine oxidase inhibitors, and narcotic and nonnarcotic pain relievers.
- Hygroton also interacts with indomethacin, steroids, digitalis, norepinephrine, some antidepressants, calcium salts, vitamin D, diazoxide, furosemide, other diuretics, sulfa drugs, fenfluramine, quinidine, and lithium.

Other:
- If this drug makes you dizzy or drowsy, do not engage in activities that require alertness.

- Avoid strenuous activity or becoming overheated in hot weather; this may cause extra loss of water from your body because of excessive perspiration.
- If you have an illness that causes diarrhea or vomiting, call your doctor.
- If you develop a sensitivity to sunlight, protect yourself with clothing and a sunscreen before exposing yourself to sunlight.
- Ask your doctor if you can take this drug early in the day to avoid getting up at night to urinate.
- Before any surgery, tell the doctor or dentist you are taking this drug.

Medical Tests:

- Your doctor may want to perform periodic laboratory tests to monitor your progress on this drug, especially if you are diabetic or have gout. He or she will also want to monitor your water-salt-potassium levels during this treatment.
- Hygroton may affect the results of some blood and urine tests, including tests for thyroid and parathyroid function.
- Any drug may affect the results and accuracy of a medical test. If a doctor recommends a medical or laboratory test for any condition, inform the doctor that you are taking this drug.

INDERAL

Ingredient(s): propranolol

Equivalent Product(s): propanolol (generic)

Used for: treatment of high blood pressure, angina, and heartbeat irregularities. It is also useful in preventing migraine headaches and additional heart attacks in heart attack patients.

Dosage Form and Strength: tablets—10 mg, 40 mg, 60 mg, 80 mg, 90 mg; capsules (sustained-release)—80 mg, 120 mg, 160 mg

Storage: Store in a tightly closed container away from light, heat, and moisture.

Before Using This Drug, Tell Your Doctor: if you have asthma or any respiratory problems, including chronic obstructive pulmonary disease, bronchitis, or emphysema; a history of heart disease or heartbeat irregularities; congestive heart failure; poor circulation in fingers and toes; hypoglycemia; diabetes; overactive thyroid gland; or kidney or liver disease. Tell your doctor about any drugs, prescription or nonprescription, you are taking and about any allergies you have or any family history of allergies.

This Drug Should Not Be Used If: you are allergic to its ingredient or have a slow heartbeat, heart block greater than first degree, cardiogenic shock, heart failure (unless it results from a condition treatable by this type of drug), bronchial asthma, bronchospasm (including that associated with respiratory allergies like hay fever), or severe chronic obstructive pulmonary disease.

How to Use: Take this drug with food. Follow your doctor's advice about when to take the drug. Try to take the drug at the same time each day. Be certain to swallow the sustained-release capsules whole; do not open, chew, or crush them. Do not stop taking this drug abruptly unless your doctor instructs you to do so.

Time Required for Drug to Take Effect: one hour, reaching a peak in three or four hours (tablets); capsules are sustained-release and thus the effects persist for longer periods of time

Missing a Dose: Take the missed dose as soon as you remember, unless you are due to take the next scheduled dose within eight hours (if you take this drug once a day) or within four hours (if you take this drug more than once a day). In that case, omit the missed dose and maintain your regular schedule. Do not double the next dose.

Symptoms of Overdose: slow and/or weak pulse, weakness, dizziness on standing up, fainting, loss of consciousness, delirium, seizures, difficult or slowed breathing, bronchospasm, clammy skin

Side Effects:

Minor and expected:
- drowsiness, dry mouth, light-headedness in upright position, cold hands and feet, fatigue

Serious adverse reactions (CALL YOUR DOCTOR):
- sore throat, fever, breathing difficulties, night cough, wheezing, nasal stuffiness, chest pain, slow pulse (less than 60 beats per minute), retention of fluids, worsening of angina, heartbeat irregularities, dizziness, fainting, depression, lethargy, sleeplessness, anxiety, nervousness, nightmares or odd dreams, confusion, behavior changes, hallucinations, slurred speech, ringing in the ears, headache, short-term memory loss, numbness or tingling of fingers

and toes, reduced sexual interest and/or ability, abdominal pain or cramping, nausea, vomiting, constipation, diarrhea, loss of appetite, urination difficulty and/or frequency, bruising, eye discomfort, dry and burning eyes, blurred vision, rash, itching, skin irritation, dry skin, sweating, changes in skin color, reversible baldness, joint pain, muscle cramps and pain

Effects of Long-Term Use: Long-term use in high doses may lead to reduced strength of heart muscle, which may increase the risk of heart failure.

Habit-Forming Possibility: none

Precautions and Suggestions:

Foods and beverages:
- No food restrictions.
- Consult your doctor before drinking alcoholic beverages because alcohol may increase the action of Inderal.

Other medicines, prescription and nonprescription:
- Inderal may interact with anesthetics and should be discontinued gradually before any surgery. Be certain your doctor, surgeon, and/or dentist knows you are taking this drug before any surgical procedure is begun.
- Nicotine in tobacco may decrease the effectiveness of this drug. Ask your doctor about smoking while taking this drug.
- Inderal may increase the effects of other high blood pressure medications, insulin and oral antidiabetics, barbiturates, narcotics, and reserpine.
- Inderal may decrease the effects of aspirin, cortisone, and other anti-inflammatory drugs. Inderal also decreases the effects of antihistamines used to treat allergies.
- Inderal may also interact with digitalis, digoxin, verapamil, nifedipine, diltiazem, monoamine oxidase inhibitors, phenothiazines, quinidine, phenytoin, chlopromazine, cimetidine, oral contraceptives, isoproterenol, norepinephrine, dopamine, dobutamine, furosemide, hydralazine, rifampin, phenobarbital, indomethacin, theophylline and other bronchodilators, thyroid hormones, epinephrine, clonidine, prazosin, and lidocaine.

Other:
- Do not stop taking this drug abruptly unless your doctor instructs you to do so.

- If this drug makes you dizzy or drowsy, do not engage in activities that require alertness, such as driving a car or operating potentially dangerous machinery.
- This drug may hide the signs of impending hypoglycemia and change the blood sugar levels in diabetics. If you are a diabetic, work with your doctor to adjust dosages of your diabetes medications to compensate for this drug.
- Do not take any nonprescription products for cough, cold, allergy, weight control, or sinus problems without checking with your doctor.

Medical Tests:

- This drug may interfere with glucose and insulin tolerance tests.
- If you are taking Inderal on a long-term basis, your doctor may want to perform blood tests to monitor your progress.
- Your doctor may want you to take your pulse each day; if it falls below 60 beats per minute, call your doctor.
- Any drug may affect the results and accuracy of a medical test. If a doctor recommends a medical or laboratory test for any condition, inform the doctor that you are taking this drug.

INDOCIN

Ingredient(s): indomethacin

Equivalent Product(s): indomethacin (generic)

Used for: relief of the symptoms of various types of arthritis as well as relief of mild to moderate pain

Dosage Form and Strength: capsules—25 mg, 50 mg; capsules (sustained-release)—75 mg; suppositories—50 mg

Storage: Store in tightly closed container away from heat and light.

Before Using This Drug, Tell Your Doctor: if you have active stomach inflammation, peptic ulcer, certain types of colitis, kidney or liver disease, urination problems, congestive heart failure, epilepsy, parkinsonism, blood-clotting or bleeding disorders, heart disease, high blood pressure, anemia, eye problems, a history of mental illness, or current or recent infection. Tell your doctor about any drugs, prescription or nonprescription, you are taking, especially anticoagulant drugs; about any allergies you have, particularly to aspirin and similar drugs; and about any family history of allergies.

This Drug Should Not Be Used If: you are allergic to its ingredient, aspirin, or any nonsteroid anti-inflammatory drug. Discuss the use of this drug with your doctor if you have active stomach or intestinal inflammation.

How to Use: Take this drug with food or immediately after meals to prevent stomach upset. If stomach irritation continues, ask your doctor if you can also take this with an antacid. Do not open, chew, or crush the sustained-release capsule. Do not take aspirin while taking Indocin. Try to take this medication on schedule.

Time Required for Drug to Take Effect: Some relief from arthritis symptoms may occur in four to 24 hours; however, it may take a few weeks for sustained relief to be achieved.

Missing a Dose: Take the missed dose as soon as you remember, unless more than an hour has passed since the missed dose was supposed to be taken. In that case, omit the missed dose and maintain the regular dosing schedule. Do not double the next dose.

Symptoms of Overdose: irritated stomach, nausea, vomiting, diarrhea, confusion, convulsions, loss of consciousness, possible bleeding from stomach or intestine

Side Effects:

Minor and expected:
- upset stomach, heartburn, drowsiness, hidden infection (because Indocin can combat or reduce fever and inflammation, its use may hide or mask an infection)

Serious adverse reactions (CALL YOUR DOCTOR):
- nausea, vomiting, diarrhea, constipation, stomach pain, abdominal pain or cramps, black stools, bleeding from stomach or intestine, yellowish discoloration of skin and whites of eyes, dizziness, headache, light-headedness, nervousness, numbness or tingling, tremor, convulsions, muscle weakness or pain, fatigue, weakness, insomnia or sleepiness, odd dreams, confusion, difficulty concentrating, depression, emotional or mental changes, congestive heart failure, rise or fall in blood pressure, heartbeat irregularities, chest pain, fluid retention, blood in urine, urination problems or changes, unusual bleeding or bruising, unexplained sore throat and fever, chills, vision problems, ringing in ears, ear pain, hearing loss, runny nose, change in taste, breathing difficulties, rash, hives, purplish discoloration of skin, increased sensitivity to sunlight, loss of hair, itching, loss of appetite, weight loss or gain, changes in blood sugar, flushing or sweating, changes in menstrual patterns, thirst, inflammation of the vagina, fainting, and loss of consciousness

Effects of Long-Term Use: eye damage

Habit-Forming Possibility: none

Precautions and Suggestions:

Foods and beverages:
- No food restrictions.
- Consult your doctor before drinking alcoholic beverages.

Other medicines, prescription and nonprescription:
- Indocin may increase the effect of anticoagulants and steroid drugs.
- Indocin should not be taken at the same time as aspirin; aspirin may interfere with the absorption of Indocin by the body.
- Indocin also may interact with anticonvulsants, sulfa drugs, oral antidiabetics, gout medicines, furosemide and thiazide diuretics, triamterene, beta blocking drugs, and lithium.

Other:
- If this drug causes you to become drowsy, do not engage in activities that require alertness, such as driving a car or operating potentially dangerous machinery.
- Because of its anti-inflammatory and fever-reducing qualities, this drug many mask the symptoms of an infection. If you suspect an infection is developing, call your doctor.
- Before any surgery, tell your doctor, surgeon, or dentist that you are taking Indocin.
- If you experience increased sensitivity to sunlight, protect yourself with clothing and a sunscreen before exposing yourself to sunlight.

Medical Tests:

- Your doctor may suggest you have periodic eye examinations while you are taking Indocin.
- Your doctor may also want to perform periodic blood and urine tests, as well as liver and kidney function tests, while you are taking this drug, to monitor your progress.
- Any drug may affect the results and accuracy of a medical test. If a doctor recommends a medical or laboratory test for any condition, inform the doctor that you are taking this drug.

INSULIN

Ingredient(s): insulin

Equivalent Product(s): Insulin is usually prescribed by type and strength, depending on each individual's needs, rather than by brand name. Discuss the advantages and disadvantages of each type and strength, based on your situation, with your doctor.

Used for: diabetics whose blood sugar level cannot be controlled by diet or weight loss

Dosage Form and Strength: injection—40 units per ml, 100 units per ml

Storage: Store unopened containers in a cool place, preferably a refrigerator. Do not freeze. Once a container has been opened, it can, and probably should, be stored at room temperature so long as the contents are used within several weeks. (Insulin injections are more comfortable if the insulin is at room temperature when it is injected.) If the container is not refrigerated, store away from strong light and high temperatures.

Before Using This Drug, Tell Your Doctor: if you have a history of kidney, liver, or thyroid disease; high fevers; or numerous infections. Tell your doctor about any drugs, prescription or nonprescription, you are taking and about any allergies you have or any family history of allergies.

This Drug Should Not Be Used If: you have had an allergic reaction to it in the past. If this is the case, you may be able to use human insulin, recently developed as an alternative to pork or beef insulin.

How to Use: First, be certain that your insulin is exactly the kind and strength your doctor ordered and that the expiration date on the container has not passed. Your doctor will show you how to inject yourself. You can use presterilized disposable needles and syringes or a glass syringe and metal needle; if you use the latter, you must sterilize them before each use. Always use the syringe that matches the strength of insulin you are taking, and always use the same type and brand of syringe to avoid making dosage mistakes.

Tip the bottle gently, end to end, to mix the insulin; do not shake the container. Check the dose in the syringe at least twice before injecting. Rub the injection site with rubbing alcohol. Avoid using cold insulin, and change the injection site every day. Your insulin injections should become a part of your daily routine so that you do not miss any doses. If you develop an illness, especially one with symptoms of diarrhea or vomiting, call your doctor. Your insulin doses will probably change during an illness.

Time Required for Drug to Take Effect: varies, depending on the type and strength of insulin being used

Missing a Dose: Try not to miss a dose. Ask your doctor what to do if you have to take a dose at an unscheduled time.

Symptoms of Overdose: hypoglycemia (low blood sugar). See "Serious adverse reactions" below.

Side Effects:

Minor and expected:
- none, if insulin dosage, diet, and physical activity are balanced and maintained

Serious adverse reactions (CALL YOUR DOCTOR):
- You should always watch carefully for three side effects: allergic reaction, hypoglycemia (low blood sugar, often called "insulin reaction"), and hyperglycemia (high blood sugar, which may lead to "diabetic coma"):
- Allergic reaction—symptoms include rash, sweating, rapid heartbeat, shortness of breath, redness or pain at site of injection.
- Hypoglycemia—symptoms include fatigue, weakness, confusion, headache, double vision, convulsions, rapid and shallow breathing, hunger, nausea, chills, tremors, paleness, moist skin, fast heartbeat, loss of consciousness.
- Hyperglycemia—symptoms include drowsiness, dim vision, and dry mouth; if prolonged, it may lead to thirst, flushing, dry skin, fruitlike breath odor, rapid heartbeat, rapid breathing, loss of appetite, nausea, vomiting, coma.

Effects of Long-Term Use: none known

Habit-Forming Possibility: none

Precautions and Suggestions:

Foods and beverages:
- Your doctor will prescribe a diet complete with meals and snacks. Follow the diet very carefully since it is balanced with your insulin doses and with a recommended physical activity schedule.

- Ask your doctor before drinking alcoholic beverages.

Other medicines, prescription and nonprescription:
- Insulin requirements may be increased by corticosteroid drugs, dextrothyroxine, danazol, epinephrine, oral contraceptives, epinephrine, dobutamine, chlorthalidone, furosemide, phenytoin, thyroid hormones, and smoking.
- The effect of insulin may be increased by monoamine oxidase inhibitors, isoniazid, aspirin, sulfa drugs, phenylbutazone, disopyramide, sulfinpyrazone, tetracycline, alcohol, and anabolic steroids.
- Insulin also may interact with some heart medications, some diuretics, beta-blocking drugs, and guanethidine.

Other:
- If you become ill, call your doctor for instructions about changing your insulin doses. An infection may cause a change in the insulin requirement. Nausea, vomiting, and diarrhea are also reasons for calling your doctor.
- Check with your doctor when planning a trip; your insulin doses may change if you change time zones.
- Exercise affects the insulin requirement on a daily basis.
- Always keep extra supplies—needles, syringes, insulin—so that you never run out.
- Carry or wear an ID that identifies you as diabetic.
- Inform your family and friends about the symptoms of insulin reaction or diabetic coma and be certain they know what to do in either event.
- At all times, carry sugar, candy, or commercial glucose to take if a hypoglycemic reaction occurs. Also keep a supply of candy in the glove compartment of your car.
- Maintain a regular eating schedule; do not skip meals or snacks.
- Be certain to tell any doctor, surgeon, or dentist that you have diabetes before undergoing any procedure.

Medical Tests:

- Your doctor will give you instructions about blood glucose and urine tests. You will perform these at home once or several times a day to monitor the amount of sugar in your blood so that you can control the balance of insulin, food, and physical activity.
- Any drug may affect the results and accuracy of a medical test. If a doctor recommends a medical or laboratory test for any condition, inform the doctor that you are taking this drug.

ISORDIL

Ingredient(s): isosorbide dinitrate

Equivalent Product(s): Dilatrate, Iso-Bid, Isonate, isosorbide dinitrate (generic), Isotrate, Onset, Sorate, Sorbide T.D., Sorbitrate

Used for: relief or prevention of chest pain of angina pectoris

Dosage Form and Strength: tablets, sublingual—2.5 mg, 5 mg, 10 mg; tablets, chewable—5 mg, 10 mg; tablets, oral—5 mg, 10 mg, 20 mg, 30 mg, 40 mg; tablets, sustained-release—40 mg (called Isordil Tembids); capsules, sustained-release—40 mg (called Isordil Tembids)

Storage: Store in a tightly closed container in a cool place away from heat, light, and moisture.

Before Using This Drug, Tell Your Doctor: if you have a history of anemia, heart attack, high blood pressure, depression, head injury, stroke, low blood pressure upon standing up, stomach or intestinal disorders, or glaucoma. Tell the doctor about any drugs, prescription or nonprescription, you are taking and about any allergies you have or any family history of allergies.

This Drug Should Not Be Used If: you are allergic to its ingredient or to similar drugs; if you have severe anemia, a recent heart attack, or a head injury. This drug should probably not be used by those with a history of stroke or a drop in blood pressure upon standing up.

How to Use: Place the sublingual tablet under your tongue or against the side of your cheek. Allow it to dissolve; do not chew or swallow it. The chewable tablets should be chewed for at least two minutes before swallowing. Do not rinse your mouth for several minutes. Take either form of these tablets at the first sign of anginal chest pain; do not wait for the pain to become severe. Then sit down and refrain from eating, drinking, or smoking while tablet is in your mouth. These forms of the drug are for immediate relief of the pain. Ask your doctor how many you can take without any resulting improvement before you should call the doctor.

The oral tablets and capsules are used to *prevent* angina pain. Take these with a full glass of water on an empty stomach. Do not open, crush, or chew the sustained-release forms; they must be swallowed whole.

Time Required for Drug to Take Effect: The effect of the sublingual and chewable forms begins in two to five minutes and lasts for one to two hours. The effect of the oral forms begins in one-half to one hour and lasts for four to six hours.

Missing a Dose: Take the missed dose as soon as you remember, unless it is within two hours of the next dose (or six hours for the sustained-release forms). In that case, omit the missed dose and return to your regular dosing schedule. Do not double the next dose.

Symptoms of Overdose: severe headache, blurred vision, dry mouth, heartbeat irregularities, warm and flushed skin, dizziness, fainting, heavy sweating, convulsions, loss of consciousness

Side Effects:

Minor and expected:
• mild headache, dizziness, flushing, light-headedness

Serious adverse reactions (CALL YOUR DOCTOR):
• severe or persistent headache, nausea, vomiting, abdominal pain, incontinence, fear, weakness, restlessness, faintness, rapid pulse, dizziness on standing up, increased chest pain, palpitations, rash, warm and flushed skin, sweating

Effects of Long-Term Use: development of tolerance to the drug; also changes in blood's hemoglobin

Habit-Forming Possibility: none

Precautions and Suggestions:

Foods and beverages:
• No food restrictions.
• Avoid alcoholic beverages.

Other medicines, prescription and nonprescription:
• Isordil may interact with drugs for high blood pressure, beta blockers, phenothiazines, drugs for glaucoma, and some antidepressants.
• The effectiveness of this drug can be affected by over-the-counter preparations for coughs, colds, asthma, allergy, and weight loss.

Other:
• If this drug makes you dizzy or drowsy, do not engage in activities that require alertness, such as driving a car or operating potentially dangerous machinery.

- If you take this drug on a regular basis, do not stop taking it suddenly. If you are to discontinue the drug, your doctor will tell you how to do so gradually.
- If you are subject to frequent bouts of diarrhea, your body may not be absorbing the sustained-release forms of this drug. Tell your doctor if this is a problem for you.
- Be certain to tell any doctor, surgeon, or dentist that you are taking Isordil before any medical, surgical, or dental procedure.

Medical Tests:

- Your doctor will probably want to perform blood cell count tests and, if you have glaucoma, eye tests to monitor your progress on this drug.
- This drug can interfere with the results of a blood test for cholesterol.
- Any drug may affect the results and accuracy of a medical test. If a doctor recommends a medical or laboratory test for any condition, inform the doctor that you are taking this drug.

KEFLEX

Ingredient(s): cephalexin

Equivalent Product(s): none

Used for: bacterial infections of the respiratory tract, middle ear, skin, bone, and urinary tract

Dosage Form and Strength: capsules—250 mg, 500 mg; tablets—1,000 mg; oral suspension—125 mg per 5 ml, 250 mg per 5 ml; pediatric suspension—100 mg per ml

Storage: Store tablets and capsules in a tightly closed container. Oral suspension should be stored in the refrigerator. After 14 days, any unused portion of the oral suspension should be discarded.

Before Using This Drug, Tell Your Doctor: if you have colitis or other intestinal disorders; a history of asthma, hay fever, or hives; bleeding disorders; diabetes; or liver or kidney disease. Tell your doctor about any drugs, prescription or nonprescription, you are taking; about any allergies you have, especially to penicillin; and about any family history of allergies.

This Drug Should Not Be Used If: you are allergic to its ingredient or to any similar antibiotics.

How to Use: Take the tablets and capsules with food or milk to prevent somach upset. If you are using the liquid form of the drug, measure it with a medical teaspoon, not an ordinary kitchen teaspoon. Ask your doctor if you can mix the liquid form with food or milk. Take at regularly spaced intervals around the clock as instructed by your doctor. Take all of the medicine prescribed even if you feel well.

Time Required for Drug to Take Effect: varies, depending on the infection; usually two to five days

Missing a Dose: Take the missed dose as soon as you remember . If you do not remember until almost time for the next dose, space that dose about halfway through the normal interval between doses. For example, if you are to take a dose at 8:00 A.M., 2:00 P.M., and 8:00 P.M., and vou remember at 7:00 P.M. that you forgot the 2:00 P.M. dose, take the missed dose at 7:00 P.M., but wait until 11:00 P.M. to take the 8:00 P.M. dose. Then return to your normal schedule. Do not skip a dose or double a dose.

Symptoms of Overdose: nausea, vomiting, abdominal cramps, diarrhea

Side Effects:

Minor and expected:
- loss of appetite, dizziness, mild diarrhea, upset stomach

Serious adverse reactions (CALL YOUR DOCTOR):
- nausea, vomiting, diarrhea, abdominal pain, indigestion, colitis, urination problems, hives, generalized itching, rash, joint pain, chest tightness, fluid retention, flushed skin, unexplained fever or sore throat, headache, dizziness, numbness or prickling, muscle cramps, vaginal discharge, breathing difficulty, sore mouth, unusual bleeding or bruising, itching in the genital and rectal areas

Effects of Long-Term Use: superinfection—that is, a second infection in addition to the infection being treated. A superinfection is caused by bacteria and other organisms that are not susceptible to or affected by the treatment being used for the original infection. Thus, these organisms, which are normally too few in number to cause problems, grow unchecked and cause a second infection that may require treatment with a different drug.

Habit-Forming Possibility: none

Precautions and Suggestions:

Foods and beverages:
- No food restrictions.
- Ask your doctor about drinking alcoholic beverages.

Other medicines, prescription and nonprescription:

- Keflex may interact with other bacteria-killing agents, probenecid, and certain diuretics.
- Keflex may increase the effects of anticoagulants.
- Kefex may increase the side effects, especially on the kidneys, of furosemide, colistin, vancomycin, polymyxin B, bumetanide, ethacrynic acid, and aminoglycoside antibiotics.

Other:

- If this drug causes you to be dizzy, do not engage in activities that require alertness, such as driving a car or operating potentially dangerous machinery.
- If this drug causes mild diarrhea, ask your doctor if you can eat yogurt. The beneficial bacteria in yogurt replace the intestine's natural beneficial bacteria that have been reduced or eliminated by Keflex.

Medical Tests:

- Your doctor may want to perform laboratory tests to monitor your progress on this drug.
- This drug may interfere with the results of some urine glucose tests a diabetic may perform at home. Ask your doctor which urine test will be accurate while you are taking this drug.
- This drug may interfere with the results of laboratory urine and blood tests.
- Any drug may affect the results and accuracy of a medical test. If a doctor recommends a medical or laboratory test for any condition, inform the doctor that you are taking this drug.

KENALOG

Ingredient(s): triamcinolone acetonide

Equivalent Product(s): Aristocort, Flutex, Kenac, triamcinolone acetonide (generic), Trymex

Used for: relief of skin inflammation, swelling, and itching symptoms caused by skin diseases

Dosage Form and Strength: ointment—0.025%, 0.1%, 0.5%; cream—0.025%, 0.1%, 0.5%; lotion—0.025%, 0.1%; aerosol—two-second spray delivers about 0.2 mg

Storage: Store away from light in a tightly closed container.

Before Using This Drug, Tell Your Doctor: if you have a fungus infection or any other infection, tuberculosis of the skin, chicken pox, shingles, herpes simplex on the skin, a perforated eardrum, diabetes, liver disease, cataract, glaucoma, osteoporosis, high blood pressure, underactive thyroid gland, myasthenia gravis, ulcer, or a circulatory system disorder. Tell your doctor if you smoke. Also, tell your doctor about any drugs, prescription or nonprescription, you are using and about any allergies you have or any family history of allergies.

This Drug Should Not Be Used If: you are allergic to its ingredient or to any steroid drugs or have a fungal infection, any other infection, tuberculosis of the skin, chicken pox, shingles, herpes simplex, ulcer, or a perforated eardrum.

How to Use: First, wash your hands and then gently wash the affected area of skin with water; pat dry. Apply the medication in a thin film; rub in lightly. Do not apply a thick layer. Do not bandage or wrap the area unless the doctor tells you to do so and shows you how. Shake the lotion well. If you are using the aerosol, do not breathe the vapors and do not pierce, puncture, or burn the can. *Do not* allow the medication to get into your eyes. Do not stop using the drug abruptly; ask the doctor how to taper off your usage.

Time Required for Drug to Take Effect: Benefits may be apparent in 24 to 48 hours. The dosage may then have to be adjusted to provide maximum benefit; this usually occurs in 4 to 10 days. It is important to adjust the dosage so that the smallest possible dose that will still achieve the desired effect is used.

Missing a Dose: Apply the missed dose as soon as you remember. However, if it is almost time for the next dose, do not apply the missed dose, but return to the original schedule. *Do not* place twice as much medication on the skin at the next dose.

Symptoms of Overdose: fatigue, increased sweating, muscle weakness, indigestion, muscle cramping, flushed face, changes in behavior

Side Effects:

Minor and expected:
- a stinging or burning sensation may occur when the medicine is applied; this is harmless

Serious adverse reactions (CALL YOUR DOCTOR):
- severe burning or stinging; itching, blistering, peeling, or any signs of irritation that were not present when you started to use Kenalog; increased hair growth; thinning of the skin; loss of skin color; signs

of infection on the skin; purplish discoloration of the skin; abnormal lines on the skin; increased sweating; muscle weakness and cramping; flushed face; indigestion; fatigue; behavior changes

Effects of Long-Term Use: weight gain, thinning of skin, easy bruising, loss of bone strength, increase in blood sugar (possibly leading to diabetes), possible development of glaucoma and cataracts

Habit-Forming Possibility: possible functional dependence in which a body function becomes dependent on the drug to do the job of the function

Precautions and Suggestions:

Foods and beverages:
* No restrictions.

Other medicines, prescription and nonprescription:
* Do not use this medication at the same time you are using another steroid medication. Elderly people can absorb a great deal of the steroid drug in this topical medication; therefore, using still another steroid medicine, oral or topical, at the same time can lead to an overdose.
* Kenalog may interact with barbiturates, sedatives, anticoagulants, glaucoma medications, thiazide diuretics, digitalis, stimulants, indomethacin, chloral hydrate, glutethimide, phenylbutazone, propranolol, aspirin, phenytoin, antihistamines, and antidiabetic drugs.
* Do not accept a vaccination while you are using this medicine.

Other:
* If you are treated by any other doctor or dentist while you are using Kenalog, be certain to tell that medical-care provider that you are using this medication.
* If you use Kenalog for an extended period of time, inform any care provider for up to two years after discontinuation that you used this drug in the past.
* This drug may decrease natural resistance to infection and reduce the body's ability to respond properly to stress, injury, or illness. Consult your doctor if there are any such changes in your health.

Medical Tests:

* Your doctor may recommend tests to monitor your progress.
* Any drug may affect the results and accuracy of a medical test. If a doctor recommends a medical or laboratory test for any condition, inform the doctor that you are taking this drug.

LANOXIN

Ingredient(s): digoxin

Equivalent Product(s): digoxin (generic)

Used for: strengthening the pumping ability of the heart and improving the rhythm of the heartbeat

Dosage Form and Strength: tablets—0.125 mg, 0.25 mg, 0.5 mg; elixir—0.05 mg per ml

Storage: Store in tightly closed container at room temperature away from light.

Before Using This Drug, Tell Your Doctor: if you have a history of any heart disorders or disease, kidney or liver disease, thyroid disorders, diabetes, lung disease, slow heart rate, Wolff-Parkinson-White syndrome, sinus node disease, any type of heart failure, low blood levels of potassium, high or low blood levels of calcium, or low blood levels of magnesium. Tell your doctor about any drugs, prescription or nonprescription, you are taking, especially digitalis, and about any allergies you have or about any family history of allergies.

This Drug Should Not Be Used If: you have certain kinds of heartbeat irregularities (ask your doctor about your condition), toxicity caused by digitalis, beriberi heart disease, or hypersensitive carotid sinus syndrome. This drug should not be used if you are allergic to its ingredient.

How to Use: Take the dose with food to prevent stomach upset. Try to take it at the same time every day. Antacids decrease the absorption of Lanoxin; therefore do not take antacids for one hour before and two hours after taking Lanoxin. If you take the liquid form of the drug or are administering it to an elderly person, use a medical teaspoon to measure the dose. An ordinary kitchen teaspoon is not accurate enough.

Time Required for Drug to Take Effect: The effect of the drug begins in about one hour and reaches a peak in six to seven hours.

Missing a Dose: Do not take the missed dose. Omit that dose and take the next dose at the regularly scheduled time. Do not double the dose. Call the doctor if you miss more than two doses in a row.

Symptoms of Overdose: nausea, vomiting, diarrhea, loss of appetite, excessive saliva, change in heartbeat, intestinal bleeding, drowsiness, headache, confusion, delirium, hallucinations, convulsions

Side Effects:

Minor and expected:
- upset stomach

Serious adverse reactions (CALL YOUR DOCTOR):
- nausea, vomiting, loss of appetite, abdominal pain, diarrhea, breast enlargement in men, skin rash, hives, changes in vision, lethargy, confusion, drowsiness, depression

Effects of Long-Term Use: development of side effects because of cumulative effects of this type of drug

Habit-Forming Possibility: none

Precautions and Suggestions:

Foods and beverages:
- Avoid eating foods high in bran fiber at the same time you take Lanoxin, which may reduce the absorption of Lanoxin from the intestine. However, bran may be eaten when you are not taking a dose of the drug.
- Ask your doctor about drinking alcoholic beverages while taking this drug.

Other medicines, prescription and nonprescription:
- The absorption of Lanoxin can be reduced by antacids, kaolin-pectin, cholestyramine, or colestipol.
- Lanoxin also may interact with diuretics, spironolactone, quinidine, quinine, procainamide, beta blockers, thyroid hormones, methimazole, propylthiouracil, calcium, reserpine, ephedrine, epinephrine, succinylcholine, some antibiotics, aminosalicylic acid, sulfasalazine, metoclopramide, anticancer drugs, insulin, hydroxychloroquine, verapamil, nifedipine, penicillamine, or steroid drugs.

Other:
- Do not discontinue medication without consulting your doctor.
- Do not change brands, including switching to a generic form of this drug, without consulting your doctor.
- Avoid over-the-counter products for coughs, colds, allergy, or weight loss.
- If you develop any other illness, especially one that causes vomiting, diarrhea, or liver effects such as yellowish discoloration of skin and whites of eyes, call your doctor; such an illness can impair the proper action of this drug.
- Before any medical or surgical procedure, tell your doctor, surgeon, or dentist that you are taking Lanoxin.

Medical Tests:

- Your doctor may want you to take your pulse daily. If it drops below 60 beats per minute, call your doctor.
- Your doctor may want to perform certain medical tests to monitor your progress on this drug.
- This drug can interfere with the results of some urine tests.
- Any drug may affect the results and accuracy of a medical test. If a doctor recommends a medical or laboratory test for any condition, inform the doctor that you are taking this drug.

LASIX

Ingredient(s): furosemide

Equivalent Product(s): furosemide (generic), SK-Furosemide

Used for: treatment of high blood pressure as well as to reduce fluid accumulation caused by conditions such as congestive heart failure, cirrhosis of the liver, or kidney disease

Dosage Form and Strength: tablets—20 mg, 40 mg, 80 mg; oral solution—10 mg per ml

Storage: Store in a tightly closed container at room temperature away from light. Exposure to light may discolor tablets. Refrigerate oral solution, but do not freeze.

Before Using This Drug, Tell Your Doctor: if you have a history of kidney or liver disease, disorder with the body's fluid-mineral balance, systemic lupus erythematosus, diarrhea bouts, heart disease, or gout. Tell your doctor about any drugs, prescription or nonprescription, you are taking and about any allergies, especially to sulfa drugs, you have or any family history of allergies.

This Drug Should Not Be Used If: you have urination problems or are allergic to its ingredient. This drug should not be used by those with hepatic coma or severe fluid-mineral imbalance until the condition is corrected.

How to Use: Take the drug with food or milk to prevent stomach upset. If you are taking the oral solution, measure it with a medical teaspoon or dropper; an ordinary kitchen teaspoon is not accurate enough. Ask your doctor if you can avoid taking a dose after 6:00 P.M. so that you do not need to get up during the night to urinate.

Time Required for Drug to Take Effect: The urine output will increase in about one hour, reach a peak in the second hour, and gradually subside in six to eight hours. Your doctor may want you to take the drug for about two weeks and then determine this drug's effectiveness in correcting your condition.

Missing a Dose: Take the missed dose as soon as you remember, unless it is almost time for your next dose. In that case, do not take the missed dose, but return to your regular dosing schedule. Do not double the next dose.

Symptoms of Overdose: weakness, lethargy, confusion, nausea, vomiting, muscle cramps, dizziness, thirst, weak and rapid pulse, drowsiness, deep sleep

Side Effects:

Minor and expected:
- frequent urination, fatigue, loss of appetite

Serious adverse reactions (CALL YOUR DOCTOR):
- muscle weakness, muscle spasm, cramps, nausea, vomiting, diarrhea, abdominal pain, constipation, yellowish discoloration of skin and whites of eyes, dizziness, blurred vision, headache, ringing in the ears, hearing loss, purplish discoloration of skin, increased sensitivity to light, rash, hives, itching, restlessness, urination problems, pain in legs

Effects of Long-Term Use: impairment of fluid-mineral balance in body tissues; possible development of diabetes-like condition in susceptible persons if fluid balance upset

Habit-Forming Possibility: none

Precautions and Suggestions:

Foods and beverages:
- Since this drug can cause potassium loss, your doctor may prescribe a diet with extra potassium. However, do not change your diet without consulting your doctor.
- Your doctor may also ask you to make changes in your intake of salt.
- Ask your doctor if you can drink alcoholic beverages while taking this drug.

Other medicines, prescription and nonprescription:
- Lasix may increase the effects of other high blood pressure medications and theophylline.

- If Lasix causes excessive potassium loss in persons also taking digitalis, digitalis poisoning may occur.
- Lasix may decrease the effects of oral diabetic drugs, insulin, and gout medications.
- Lasix also may interact with digoxin, lithium, some antibiotics, barbiturates, narcotics, corticosteroid drugs, aspirin or other salicylates, indomethacin, ibuprofen, naproxen, metolazone, norepinephrine, tubocurarine, succinylcholine, and phenytoin.

Other:

- The oral form of Lasix contains a dye called *tartrazine* that may cause an allergic reaction in susceptible persons.
- If you have any illness that causes vomiting, diarrhea, or other water loss, call your doctor.
- If Lasix causes an increased sensitivity to sunlight, wear protective clothing and an effective sunscreen when exposed to sunlight.
- If this drug causes drowsiness or dizziness, do not engage in activities that require alertness, such as driving a car or operating potentially dangerous equipment.
- Do not take any over-the-counter product for coughs, colds, allergy, or sinus problems without discussing it with your doctor.
- Before any medical or surgical procedure, tell your doctor, surgeon, or dentist that you are taking Lasix.

Medical Tests:

- Your doctor may want to perform periodic tests, especially for potassium blood levels, to monitor your progress on this drug.
- Any drug may affect the results and accuracy of a medical test. If a doctor recommends a medical or laboratory test for any condition, inform the doctor that you are taking this drug.

LINDANE (GENERIC)

Ingredient(s): gamma benzene hexachloride

Equivalent Product(s): Kwell, Scabene

Used for: treatment of head and crab lice and their eggs. Cream and lotion forms also are used to treat scabies.

Dosage Form and Strength: cream—1%; lotion—1%; shampoo—1%

Storage: Store all forms of this product at room temperature.

Before Using This Drug, Tell Your Doctor: if you have any allergies. Also tell your doctor about any medication, prescription or non-prescription, you are taking.

This Drug Should Not Be Used If: you are allergic to its ingredient

How to Use:

- *Shampoo*: Wash hair over sink rather than in bath or shower, because less of the body is exposed to the shampoo and therefore less lindane is absorbed though the skin. Apply two tablespoons of shampoo to your dry hair. Add small quantities of water and work into hair and skin until good lather forms. Do not allow shampoo to get into your eyes or mouth. Continue shampooing for four minutes. Rinse the hair well with water. Towel and comb with a fine-tooth comb to remove the nits (eggs). You should not have to repeat the treatment unless you find living lice seven days later. Do not use the shampoo more than twice. Do not use it as a routine shampoo.
- *Cream and lotion*: To treat for lice, apply enough to cover thinly the entire affected area. Rub the medicine into the skin and hair and leave it on for eight to 12 hours. Then wash thoroughly. You usually will not have to apply a second treatment unless you see living lice after seven days.
- *For scabies*: Apply a thin coating of the medicine to dry skin all over your body from the neck down. Rub it in thoroughly. Leave it on for eight to 12 hours and then remove the medicine by washing thoroughly. One application is usually all that is needed.

Time Required for Drug to Take Effect: shampoo, four minutes; cream and lotion, eight to 12 hours

Missing a Dose: not applicable

Symptoms of Overdose: This product can penetrate the skin and have an effect on the central nervous system. There have been reports of seizures following the use of this drug, but it has not been definitely proved that the drug was the cause. Studies have shown that potential adverse effects of this medication may be greater in young children and possibly in very elderly persons. Discuss the use of this drug with your doctor.

Side Effects:

Minor and expected:
- none

Serious adverse reactions (CALL YOUR DOCTOR):
- possible seizures, skin rash, itching, burning

Effects of Long-Term Use: not applicable

Habit-Forming Possibility: not applicable

Precautions and Suggestions:

Foods and beverages:
- Not applicable.

Other medicines, prescription and nonprescription:
- No restrictions.

Other:
- Do not take a hot bath or shampoo immediately before treatment with lindane.
- Do not apply to the face; avoid getting the product in the eyes.
- Do not use more than the amount prescribed.
- This medication is poisonous if swallowed or absorbed through the skin; make sure you rinse it off thoroughly after the prescribed treatment time. Keep this medication out of the reach of children.
- Do not use lindane if your scalp and neck have open sores. Call your doctor for advice.
- If one person within your household has lice, all family members except pregnant women and infants should be treated for lice. All sexual contacts should be treated as well.
- After shampooing and rinsing the hair, sometimes an additional vinegar rinse will loosen the nits (eggs) so that you can comb them out.
- Be certain to clean hairbrushes and combs with lindane and to launder hats, clothing, and bedding thoroughly.

Medical Tests:

- Not applicable.

LOPRESSOR

Ingredient(s): metoprolol tartrate

Equivalent Product(s): none

Used for: treatment of high blood pressure, treatment of suspected or definite heart attack, and prevention of heart attacks in certain heart attack patients

Dosage Form and Strength: tablets—50 mg, 100 mg

Storage: Store in a tightly closed container at room temperature away from light and moisture.

Before Using This Drug, Tell Your Doctor: if you have athsma or any respiratory problems, including chronic obstructive pulmonary disease, bronchitis, or emphysema; a history of heart disease; congestive heart failure; poor circulation in fingers and toes; hypoglycemia; diabetes; overactive thyroid gland; or kidney or liver disease. Tell your doctor about any drugs, prescription and nonprescription, you are taking and about any allergies you have or any family history of allergies.

This Drug Should Not Be Used If: you are allergic to its ingredient or have slow heartbeat, heart block greater than first degree, cardiogenic shock, heart failure (unless it results from a condition treatable by this drug), low blood pressure, bronchial asthma, bronchospasm (including that associated with respiratory allergies like hay fever), or severe chronic obstructive pulmonary disease.

How to Use: Take this drug with food. Follow your doctor's advice about when to take the drug. Try to take the drug at the same time every day. Do not stop taking the drug abruptly unless your doctor instructs you to do so.

Time Required for Drug to Take Effect: one hour, reaching a peak in three to four hours, and persisting for 24 hours. Consistent use for several weeks may be necessary to detemine Lopressor's effectiveness in treating your condition.

Missing a Dose: Take the missed dose as soon as you remember, unless you are due to take the next scheduled dose within eight hours if you take the drug once a day or within four hours if you take the drug more than once a day. In that case, omit the missed dose and maintain your regular schedule. Do not double the next dose.

Symptoms of Overdose: slow and/or weak pulse, weakness, dizziness on standing up, fainting, loss of consciousness, delirium, seizures, difficult or slowed breathing, bronchospasm, clammy skin

Side Effects:

Minor and expected:
- drowsiness, dry mouth, cold hands and feet, clammy skin

Serious adverse reactions (CALL YOUR DOCTOR):
- sore throat, fever, light-headedness in upright position, breathing difficulties, night cough, wheezing, nasal stuffiness, chest pain, slow pulse (less than 60 beats per minute), retention of fluids, worsening of chest pain, heartbeat irregularities, dizziness, fainting, depression, lethargy, sleeplessness, anxiety, nervousness,

nightmares or odd dreams, confusion, behavior changes, hallucinations, slurred speech, ringing in the ears, headache, short-term
memory loss, numbness or tingling of fingers and toes, reduced
sexual interest and/or ability, abdominal pain or cramping, nausea,
vomiting, constipation, diarrhea, loss of appetite, urination difficulties and/or frequency, bruising, eye discomfort, dry and burning eyes, blurred vision, rash, itching, skin irritation, dry skin,
sweating, changes in skin color, reversible baldness, joint pain,
muscle cramps and pain

Effects of Long-Term Use: Long-term use in high doses may lead to
reduced strength of heart muscle, which may increase the risk of heart
failure.

Habit-Forming Possibility: none

Precautions and Suggestions:

Foods and beverages:
- No food restrictions.
- Consult your doctor before drinking alcoholic beverages because
alcohol may increase the action of Lopressor.

Other medicines, prescription and nonprescription:
- Lopressor may interact with anesthetics and should be discontinued gradually before any surgery. Be certain your doctor,
surgeon, or dentist knows you are taking this drug before any
surgical procedure is begun.
- Nicotine in tobacco may decrease the effectiveness of this drug.
Ask your doctor about smoking while taking this drug.
- Lopressor may increase the effects of other high blood pressure
medications, insulin and oral diabetes drugs, barbiturates, narcot-
ics, and reserpine.
- Lopressor may decrease the effects of aspirin, cortisone, and other
anti-inflamatory drugs. Lopressor also decreases the effects of
antihistamines used to treat allergies.
- Lopressor may also interact with digitalis, digoxin, verapamil
(Isoptin), nifedipine (Procardia), diltiazem, quinidine, phenytoin
(Dilantin), chlorpromazine, phenothiazines, monoamine oxidase
inhibitors, cimetidine (Tagamet), oral contraceptives, furosemide
(Lasix), hydralazine, rifampin, phenobarbital, indomethacin, prazosin, thyroid drugs, lidocaine, isoproterenol, norepinephrine,
dopamine, dobutamine, epinephrine, theophyllines and other
bronchodilators, and clonidine.

Other:

- Do not stop taking this drug abruptly unless the doctor instructs you to do so. This drug must be discontinued gradually.
- If this drug makes you dizzy or drowsy, do not engage in activities that require alertness, such as driving a car or operating potentially dangerous equipment.
- This drug may hide signs of impending hypoglycemia and change the blood sugar levels in diabetics. If you are diabetic, work with your doctor to adjust dosages of your diabetes medications to compensate for this drug.
- Do not take any over-the-counter products for cough, colds, allergies, or sinus problems without discussing it with your doctor.

Medical Tests:

- This drug may interfere with glucose and insulin tolerance tests as well as other laboratory tests.
- If you are taking Lopressor on a long-term basis, your doctor may want to perform blood tests to monitor your progress.
- Your doctor may want you to take your pulse each day; if it drops below 60 beats per minute, call your doctor.
- Any drug may affect the results and accuracy of a medical test. If a doctor recommends a medical or laboratory test for any condition, inform the doctor that you are taking this drug.

MINIPRESS

Ingredient(s): prazosin

Equivalent Product(s): none

Used for: treating high blood pressure

Dosage Form and Strength: capsules—1 mg, 2 mg, 5 mg

Storage: Store in a tightly closed container at room temperature away from light.

Before Using This Drug, Tell Your Doctor: if you have heart disease, angina, impaired circulation, kidney disease, systemic lupus erythematosus, or mental depression. Tell the doctor about any drugs, prescription or nonprescription, you are taking and about any allergies you have or any family history of allergies.

This Drug Should Not Be Used If: you are allergic to its ingredient.

How to Use: Take with food or water. The very first dose may cause fainting; therefore, it is often recommended that this dose be taken at bedtime. Try to take the drug at the same time every day.

Time Required for Drug to Take Effect: The effect of the drug begins in one-half hour and peaks in two to three hours. Your doctor may want you to use Minipress on a consistent basis for four to six weeks to determine if this drug is effective for your condition.

Missing a Dose: Take the missed dose as soon as you remember, unless it is almost time for your next dose. In that case, do not take the missed dose, but return to your regular dosing schedule. Do not double the next dose.

Symptoms of Overdose: extreme dizziness or light-headedness in upright position, rapid heartbeat, headache, flushed skin, weak pulse, extreme weakness, cold and sweaty skin, loss of consciousness

Side Effects:

Minor and expected:
- drowsiness, lack of energy, loss of appetite, headache, nausea, weakness, pounding heartbeat

Serious adverse reactions (CALL YOUR DOCTOR):
- dizziness or light-headedness upon rising from a lying or sitting position, fainting, irregular heartbeat, blurred vision, mental depression, vomiting, constipation, diarrhea, abdominal pain, frequent urination, nervousness, impotence, constant erection, inability to control urination, dry mouth, nasal congestion, hallucinations, loss of hair, rapid weight gain, swelling of feet or legs, ringing in the ears, tingling in fingers or toes, nosebleeds, excessive sweating, rash, itching, vivid dreams, chest pain, difficulty in breathing or urinating, possible low body temperature

Effects of Long-Term Use: none known

Habit-Forming Possibility: none

Precautions and Suggestions:

Foods and beverages:
- No food restrictions, although your doctor may recommend a low-sodium or reducing diet depending on your situation.
- Your doctor may tell you to avoid alcoholic beverages.

Other medicines, prescription and nonprescription:
- Minipress may interact with other high blood pressure drugs, nitroglycerine, phenothiazines, some antidepressants, amphetamines, and alcohol.

Other:

- If this drug makes you drowsy or dizzy, do not engage in activities that require alertness, such as driving a car or using potentially dangerous equipment.
- Fainting may occur after the first dose of Minipress; do not drive or operate machinery for four hours after the first dose.
- Avoid becoming overheated (strenuous exercise, hot tubs, hot showers, saunas) to prevent light-headedness and fainting.
- Do not take any over-the-counter products for cough, cold, allergy, weight loss, or sinus problems without talking to your doctor.
- Do not stop taking this drug abruptly without talking to your doctor.
- Tell any doctor, surgeon, or dentist you are taking this medication before any medical, surgical, or dental procedure.

Medical Tests:

- Your doctor may want to perform periodic tests to monitor your progress on this drug, especially blood pressure tests in a lying, sitting, and standing position.
- Any drug may affect the results and accuracy of a medical test. If a doctor recommends a medical or laboratory test for any condition, inform the doctor that you are taking this drug.

MONISTAT-7

Ingredient(s): miconazole nitrate

Equivalent Product(s): none

Used for: treatment of fungal infections of the vagina

Dosage Form and Strength: vaginal cream—2% with applicator; vaginal suppositories—100 mg with applicator

Storage: Store in a tightly closed container at room temperature.

Before Using This Drug, Tell Your Doctor: if you have diabetes or a history of vaginal infections, particularly if they were resistant to treatment. Tell your doctor about any drugs, prescription or nonprescription, you are taking and about any allergies you have or any family history of allergies.

This Drug Should Not Be Used If: you are allergic to its ingredient. You should not use this drug for a different infection later on; it may be caused by a different organism and thus require another medication.

How to Use: Carefully read the instuctions accompanying the medication package. Wash the genital area before inserting cream or suppository. Insert high into the vagina. If you begin to menstruate while completing this therapy session, continue to use Monistat-7 through your period. Use this medication for the entire time prescribed by your doctor even if you feel well and your symptoms disappear.

Time Required for Drug to Take Effect: Usually a seven-day course of therapy is sufficient, but it may be repeated if necessary.

Missing a Dose: Insert the missed dose as soon as you remember, unless you do not remember until the following day. In that case, return to your regular dosing schedule. Do not double the next dose.

Symptoms of Overdose: none reported

Side Effects:

Minor and expected:
- mild burning, itching, or irritation at site of insertion or in vagina

Serious adverse reactions (CALL YOUR DOCTOR):
- increased local burning, itching, or irritation; lower abdominal cramps; headache; skin rash; hives

Effects of Long-Term Use: This drug is not prescribed for long-term use.

Habit-Forming Possibility: none

Precautions and Suggestions:

Foods and beverages:
- No restrictions.

Other medicines, prescription and nonprescription:
- No interactions reported if used according to directions.

Other:
- To prevent reinfection, avoid sexual intercourse or ask partner to use a condom until course of treatment is completed. Ask your doctor if your partner should also be treated.
- To avoid staining of clothes, use a sanitary napkin or panty liner during treatment.
- Wear cotton underpants, rather than synthetic material, to allow for absorption and exchange of air that nonporous, synthetic fabrics do not permit.
- If there is no improvement in your condition after several days of treatment, call your doctor.

Medical Tests:

- Your doctor may want to take cultures and smears of vaginal secretions to determine the cause of your infection or reinfection.
- Any drug may affect the results and accuracy of a medical test. If a doctor recommends a medical or laboratory test for any condition, inform the doctor that you are taking this drug.

MYCOSTATIN

Ingredient(s): nystatin

Equivalent Product(s): Korostatin, Nilstat, nystatin (generic)

Used for: treatment of yeast and fungal infections

Dosage Form and Strength: tablets—500,000 units; oral suspension—100,000 units per ml; cream or ointment—100,000 units per gram; vaginal tablets—100,000 units; powder—100,000 units per gram

Storage: Store all but vaginal tablet at room temperature. Refrigerate the vaginal tablet. (The Korostatin vaginal tablet does not need refrigeration.)

Before Using This Drug, Tell Your Doctor: about any drug, prescription or nonprescription, you are taking and about any known allergies or any family history of allergies.

This Drug Should Not Be Used If: you are allergic to its ingredient.

How to Use:

- *Tablets*: Take as directed. Continue taking tablets for at least 48 hours after the infection clears up.
- *Cream or ointment*: Apply medicine to affected areas after cleaning the areas, unless instructed otherwise by your doctor. Continue using for one week after the infection has disappeared. Do not use in eyes.
- *Oral suspension*: If you are treating an infection in the mouth, hold the medicine in your mouth and rinse it around as long as possible before swallowing. Shake the container well before using. Continue taking the medicine for at least 48 hours after the infection is gone.
- *Vaginal tablets*: With accompanying applicator, insert one tablet high into the vagina daily. Use all the medication on a continuous basis, even during a menstrual period.

Time Required for Drug to Take Effect: varies, depending on infection; usually one to three weeks

Missing a Dose: Take the dose when you remember and then return to the regular dosing schedule. If you remember just before the next dose is due, wait until that time, take the dose, and continue the regular schedule. Do not double the next dose.

Symptoms of Overdose: There is little possibility of overdosing, but nausea, vomiting, stomachache, and diarrhea have occurred in those taking large doses.

Side Effects:

Minor and expected:
* none

Serious adverse reactions (CALL YOUR DOCTOR):
* nausea, vomiting, stomachache, diarrhea, skin irritation or burning (ointment or cream)

Effects of Long-Term Use: none

Habit-Forming Possibility: not applicable

Precautions and Suggestions:

Foods and beverages:
* No restrictions.

Other medicines, prescription and nonprescription:
* No interactions.

Other:
* The powder form is best for wet, weeping sores.
* The oral suspension does not have to be refrigerated.
* Always complete the full course of medication, even if you seem well.
* Avoid sexual intercourse if you are treating a vaginal infection. Also, use a sanitary napkin to prevent stained clothing.

Medical Tests:

* No known interferences.
* Your doctor may want to perform diagnostic tests if there is no response to this drug.
* A persistent yeast infection may be a sign of undiagnosed diabetes, and your doctor may test for this.
* Any drug may affect the results and accuracy of a medical test. If a doctor recommends a medical or laboratory test for any condition, inform the doctor that you are taking this drug.

NAPROSYN

Ingredient(s): naproxen

Equivalent Product(s): Anaprox

Used for: relief of mild to moderate pain and treatment of painful menstruation, certain forms of arthritis, bursitis, tendinitis, gout, and ankylosing spondylitis

Dosage Form and Strength: tablets—250 mg, 375 mg, 500 mg

Storage: Store in tightly closed container away from heat and light.

Before Using This Drug, Tell Your Doctor: if you have kidney or liver disease; stomach or intestinal problems, including ulcers; bleeding problems; heart disease; high blood pressure; anemia; diabetes; epilepsy; parkinsonism; or a history of a sensitivity to aspirin. Tell your doctor about any drugs, prescription or nonprescription, you are taking and about any allergies you have, especially to aspirin, sulindac, ibuprofen, fenoprofen, naproxen, indomethacin, tolmetin, zomepirac, mefenamic acid, meclofenamate, or piroxicam. Also tell your doctor about any family history of allergies.

This Drug Should Not Be Used If: you are allergic to aspirin or to any nonsteroidal anti-inflammatory drugs (listed at the end of the preceding paragraph), including the ingredient in this medication. This drug should be used with caution by those who have liver or kidney disease, a bleeding disorder, an active ulcer, or ulcerative colitis.

How to Use: Take with food, especially if stomach upset occurs.

Time Required for Drug to Take Effect: one to two hours, reaching a peak in two to four hours. It may take one to two weeks before significant improvement is noticeable.

Missing a Dose: Take the missed dose as soon as you remember, unless it is almost time for the next dose. In that case, omit the missed dose and return to your regular dosing schedule. Do not double the next dose.

Symptoms of Overdose: stomach upset, nausea, vomiting, diarrhea

Side Effects:

Minor and expected:
- mild stomach upset and/or cramping, drowsiness, heartburn, bloating, gas, dry mouth, loss of appetite, dizziness, headache, constipation, mild diarrhea, nervousness

Serious adverse reactions (CALL YOUR DOCTOR):
- severe stomach upset, nausea, vomiting, or diarrhea; abdominal pain; black, tarry stools; rectal bleeding; nosebleeds; mouth sores; severe headache; yellowish discoloration of skin and whites of eyes; tremor; convulsions; muscle pain or weakness; fatigue; lethargy; numbness, prickling, and tingling; nerve disorders; sleepiness or sleeplessness; depression; confusion; behavior changes; fall or rise in blood pressure; changes in heartbeat; fluid retention; chest pain; blood in urine; problems with urination; blood disorders; purplish discoloration of skin; bruising; anemia; changes in vision; irritated eyes; sensitivity to light; loss of color vision (reversible when drug is stopped); ringing in the ears; hearing loss; ear pain; stuffy nose; changes in taste; breathing difficulty; rash, itching; baldness; aggravation of epilepsy and parkinsonism; changes in blood sugar levels and increased need for insulin in diabetics; increased blood potassium levels; flushing or sweating; menstrual disorders; vaginal bleeding; vaginal infection; unexplained sore throat and fever; chills; thirst; fainting; sore tongue; breast changes in men and women

Effects of Long-Term Use: may cause changes in the eyes or kidney

Habit-Forming Possibility: none

Precautions and Suggestions:

Foods and beverages:
- No food restrictions.
- Consult your doctor before consuming alcoholic beverages with this drug.

Other medicines, prescription and nonprescription:
- Avoid aspirin while using this drug.
- Avoid antacids containing large amounts of sodium.
- Naposyn may interact with anticonvulsants, phenobarbital, sulfa drugs, diuretics, beta blockers, diabetes medications, lithium, anticoagulant drugs, other anti-inflammatory drugs, other arthritis or gout medications, and aspirin.

Other:
- If this drug causes drowsiness, dizziness, or blurred vision, do not engage in activities that require alertness, such as driving or operating potentially dangerous machinery.
- Because of its anti-inflammatory and fever-reducing qualities, this drug may mask the symptoms of an infection. If you suspect an infection is developing, call your doctor.

- Before any medical treatment, including dental treatment, tell your health-care provider that you are taking this drug.

Medical Tests:

- Your doctor may want to conduct periodic liver and kidney function tests, blood tests, and eye and hearing examinations.
- Naprosyn may interfere with the results of some laboratory tests; be certain to remind your doctor or lab technician that you are taking Naprosyn when you are tested.

NITROGLYCERIN (GENERIC)

Ingredient(s): nitroglycerin

Equivalent Product(s): Ang-O-Span, Klavikordal, N-G-C, Niong, Nitro-Bid, Nitrocap, Nitradisc, Nitro-Dur, Nitroglyn, Nitrol, Nitrolin, Nitro-Long, Nitronet, Nitrong, Nitrospan, Nitrostat, Susadrin, Transderm-Nitro, Trates

Used for: prevention and management of angina pectoris

Dosage Form and Strength: tablets, sublingual—0.15 mg, 0.3 mg, 0.4 mg, 0.6 mg; tablets, transmucosal—1 mg, 2 mg, 3 mg; tablets, sustained-release—2.6 mg, 6.5 mg, 9 mg; capsules, sustained-release—2.5 mg, 6.5 mg, 9 mg; ointment—2%; transdermal system—2.5 mg/24 hours, 5 mg/24 hours, 7.5 mg/24 hours, 10 mg/24 hours, 15 mg/24 hours

Storage: All forms of nitroglycerin should be stored in tightly closed containers away from heat, extreme cold, and moisture. The sublingual tablets, ointment, and transdermal patches should always be stored in their original containers. The sublingual tablets should not be stored in a metal or plastic bottle, but should remain in their original glass container, and they should not be stored in the refrigerator or bathroom. Do not keep cotton or paper (such as label instructions) inside the container.

Before Using This Drug, Tell Your Doctor: if you have a history of anemia, heart attack, high blood pressure, depression, head injury, stroke, low blood pressure on standing up, stomach or intestinal disorders, or glaucoma. Tell the doctor about any drugs, prescription or nonprescription, you are taking and about any allergies you have or any family history of allergies.

This Drug Should Not Be Used If: you are allergic to its ingredient or to similar drugs; if you have severe anemia, a recent heart attack, or a head injury. This drug should probably not be used by those with a history of stroke or a drop in blood pressure on standing up.

How to Use:

- *Sublingual and transmucosal tablets*: Place the sublingual tablet under your tongue. Allow it to dissolve; do not chew or swallow it. The transmucosal form is taken the same way, except it is placed between the lip and gum above the upper incisor teeth. Take either form of these tablets at the first sign of anginal chest pain; do not wait for the pain to become severe. Then sit down and refrain from eating, drinking, or smoking while tablet is in your mouth. Do not rinse your mouth afterward. These forms are for immediate relief of pain. Ask your doctor how many you can take without any resulting improvement before calling him or her. As a preventive precaution, take a sublingual tablet five or ten minutes before an activity that usually causes an anginal attack; for example, heavy exercise, exposure to extreme cold, or emotional stress.
- *Oral tablets and capsules*: These are used to prevent angina pain. Take them with a full glass of water on an empty stomach. Do not open, crush, or chew the sustained-release form; they must be swallowed whole.
- *Ointment*: Use the package's applicator to measure the ointment dose. Remove the previous dose before applying the new dose and then apply the new dose to a different site on the skin. Spread the ointment in a smooth, thin, even layer, covering about the same amount of skin each time. Do not rub or massage the ointment into the skin. Use rubber or plastic gloves to apply the ointment and do not let the ointment come into contact with other parts of the body. Do not cover the ointment unless instructed to do so by your doctor.
- *Transdermal patch*: This should be applied to a hairless or clean-shaven area, but avoid scars or wounds. Select a place that is not involved in excessive movement (such as the chest). If a patch becomes dislodged, throw it away and replace it. Always apply a new patch before removing the old one so as to maintain continuous drug therapy, and always select a new site for each new patch. You can bathe, shower, or swim with a patch in place. Do not cut or trim a patch; this changes the dose of medication you receive.

Time Required for Drug to Take Effect: The effect of the sublingual or transmucosal forms begins in one-half to three minutes and lasts for about 20 minutes. The sustained-release forms become active in about 30 minutes, and the effect lasts for about eight to 12 hours. The ointment and transdermal forms are not to be used for immediate relief, but to prevent anginal pain; they work more slowly.

Missing a Dose: This issue does not apply to the sublingual or transmucosal forms of nitroglycerin; they are used as needed for pain. If you miss a dose of the sustained-release or topical (ointment or transdermal) form, take the missed dose as soon as you remember, unless it is more than halfway through the normal interval between doses. In that case, do not take the missed dose, but return to your regular dosing schedule. Do not double the next dose.

Symptoms of Overdose: severe pounding headache, blurred vision, dry mouth, heartbeat irregularities, warm and flushed skin, dizziness, fainting, heavy sweating, convulsions, loss of consciousness

Side Effects:

Minor and expected:
- mild headache, dizziness, flushing, light-headedness. Sublingual and transmucosal forms cause a burning, tingling sensation at site of application; this is one way to tell that the tablet is still potent.

Serious adverse reactions (CALL YOUR DOCTOR):
- severe or persistent headache, nausea, vomiting, abdominal pain, incontinence, fear, weakness, restlessness, fainting, rapid pulse, dizziness on standing up, increased chest pain, palpitations, rash, (if the rash occurs with the transdermal patch, the rash could be a reaction to the patch material and not to the nitroglycerin—ask your doctor about this), warm and flushed skin, muscle twitching, paleness, sweating

Effects of Long-Term Use: development of tolerance to the drug; also, changes in blood's hemoglobin

Habit-Forming Possibility: none

Precautions and Suggestions:

Foods and beverages:
- No food restrictions.
- Avoid alcoholic beverages.

Other medicines, prescription and nonprescription:
- Nitroglycerin may interact with drugs for high blood pressure and glaucoma, beta blockers, phenothiazines, and some antidepressants.
- The effectiveness of this drug can be affected by over-the-counter (nonprescription) preparations for coughs, colds, asthma, allergy, and weight loss.

Other:
- If this drug makes you dizzy or drowsy, do not engage in activities that require alertness, such as driving a car or operating potentially dangerous machinery.
- If you take nitroglycerin on a regular basis, do not stop taking it suddenly. If you are to discontinue the drug, your doctor will tell you how to do so gradually.
- If you are subject to frequent bouts of diarrhea, your body may not be absorbing the sustained-release forms of this drug. Tell your doctor if this is a problem for you.
- Be certain to tell any doctor, surgeon, or dentist that you are taking nitroglycerin before any medical, surgical, or dental procedure.

Medical Tests:

- Your doctor will probably want to perform blood cell count tests and, if you have glaucoma, eye tests to monitor your progress on this drug.
- This drug can interfere with the results of a blood test for cholesterol.
- Any drug may affect the results and accuracy of a medical test. If a doctor recommends a medical or laboratory test for any condition, inform the doctor that you are taking this drug.

PENICILLIN V (GENERIC)

Ingredient(s): penicillin V

Equivalent Product(s): numerous generic equivalents

Used for: treating bacterial infections including infections in the middle ear, respiratory tract, skin, and gums

Dosage Form and Strength: tablets—125 mg, 250 mg, 500 mg; oral solution—125 mg per 5 ml, 250 mg per 5 ml

Storage: Store the oral solution in the refrigerator and use it within 14 days; discard any unused portion after that time. Store the tablets in a tightly closed, light-resistant container in a cool place (below 85 degrees Fahrenheit).

Before Using This Drug, Tell Your Doctor: if you have ever had an allergic or asthmatic reaction to a penicillin drug or to any other antibiotics. Also, tell your doctor if you are allergic by nature or have ever had asthma, hay fever, hives, skin rashes, or any other allergic reactions to anything. Inform your doctor if you have ever been diagnosed as having liver or kidney problems. Be sure to tell your doctor about any drugs, prescription or nonprescription, you are using.

This Drug Should Not Be Used If: you are allergic to penicillin or have previously had an allergic reaction to any form of penicillin.

How to Use: Take the medicine as directed by your doctor, usually at evenly spaced intervals around the clock. The drug can be taken with or without food. If you are using the oral solution, shake the container thoroughly and measure with a medical teaspoon. Take each dose with a full glass of water, not fruit juice or carbonated beverage. The oral solution and the tablets (crushed) can be mixed with milk or water if given to an elderly person. If you do this, you must be certain the person swallows the entire drink to receive the full dose of medicine. Take the full amount of medication until it is gone, even if you seem and feel well.

Time Required for Drug to Take Effect: varies, depending on the illness being treated; usually two to five days

Missing a Dose: Take the missed dose immediately. If it is almost time for the next dose, wait to take the next dose until about halfway through the regular interval between doses. For example, if you are to take a dose at 8:00 A.M., 2:00 P.M., and 8:00 P.M., and you remember at 7:00 P.M. that you forgot the 2:00 P.M. dose, take the missed dose at 7:00 P.M. but wait until about 11:00 P.M. to take the 8:00 P.M. dose. Then return to your regular schedule at 2:00 A.M. Do not skip a dose or double the dose.

Symptoms of Overdose: possible severe and persistent nausea, vomiting, and/or diarrhea

Side Effects:

Minor and expected:
• diarrhea, nausea

Serious adverse reactions (CALL YOUR DOCTOR):
- hives, itching (especially in the genital or anal area), or skin rash; difficult breathing; fever; joint pain; sore throat; dark-colored tongue; yellow-green stools; sores in the mouth; severe and persistent nausea, vomiting, or diarrhea; unusual fatigue; confusion; depression; convulsions

Effects of Long-Term Use: superinfection—that is, a second infection in addition to the infection being treated. A superinfection is caused by bacteria and other organisms that are not susceptible to or affected by the drug being used to treat the original infection. Thus, these organisms, which are normally too few in number to cause problems, grow unchecked and cause a second infection that may require treatment with a different drug.

Habit-Forming Possibility: none

Precautions and Suggestions:

Foods and beverages:
- No restrictions.

Other medicines, prescription and nonprescription:
- Penicillin V may interact with other antibiotics, particularly erythromycin, tetracyline, and neomycin. Be certain your doctor is told about any other antibiotics you are taking.
- Penicillin V may also decrease the effectiveness of oral contraceptives.
- Penicillin V also interacts with probenecid.

Other:
- If mild diarrhea is a side effect, ask your doctor if you can eat yogurt. The beneficial bacteria in yogurt replace the intestine's natural beneficial bacteria that have been reduced or eliminated by the penicillin.
- Do not use this drug beyond the expiration date on its label.

Medical Tests:

- Your doctor may recommend blood tests and liver and kidney function tests during treatment with this drug in order to monitor your progress.
- Any drug may affect the results and accuracy of a medical test. If a doctor recommends a medical or laboratory test for any condition, inform the doctor that you are taking this drug.

PHENOBARBITAL (GENERIC)

Ingredient(s): phenobarbital

Equivalent Product(s): Barbita, Luminal Ovoids, PBR/12, Sedadrops, SK-Phenobarbital, Solfoton

Used for: control of convulsions or seizures, relief of anxiety or tension, and as a sleeping aid

Dosage Form and Strength: tablets—8 mg, 15 mg, 16 mg, 30 mg, 32 mg, 65 mg, 100 mg; capsules—16 mg; capsules, timed-release—65 mg; drops—16 mg per ml; liquid—15 mg per 5 ml; elixir—20 mg per 5 ml

Storage: Store capsules and tablets in dry, tightly closed container at room temperature. Store liquid in tightly closed and dark-colored container.

Before Using This Drug, Tell Your Doctor: if you have chronic lung disease, diabetes, epilepsy, liver or kidney disease, overactive thyroid, disorders of the adrenal glands, anemia, or porphyria (an inherited disease characterized by sensitivity to sunlight and liver involvement). Also, tell your doctor about any drugs, prescription or nonprescription, you are taking and about any allergies you have or any family history of allergies.

This Drug Should Not Be Used If: you are allergic to its ingredient or to any barbiturate or if you have liver or kidney disease, respiratory disease, or porphyria. This drug should not be used by anyone with a previous addiction to sedatives or hypnotics or a history of drug abuse, depression, or suicidal tendencies.

How to Use: Take phenobarbital with food or a full glass of water. Measure the liquid forms with a medical teaspoon. You can also crush the tablets or open the regular capsule and place the drug in food, but you must eat all the food in order to receive the full dose. You must not open the timed-release capsule; it must be swallowed whole.

Time Required for Drug to Take Effect: about one hour

Missing a Dose: If you remember within an hour of the regular dosage time, take the missed dose and then return to the regular dosing schedule. If more than an hour has passed, do not take the missed dose, but return to the regular schedule. Do not double the next dose.

Symptoms of Overdose: confusion, slurred speech, drowsiness, clumsiness, reduced urine volume, staggering walk, slow and shallow breathing, weak and rapid pulse, cold and sweaty skin, deep sleep, lowered body temperature, eventually coma

Side Effects:

Minor and expected:
* drowsiness, sleepiness, a hangover feeling, dizziness, nausea, vomiting, diarrhea, headache, constipation, muscle pain, joint pain

Serious adverse reactions (CALL YOUR DOCTOR):
* sore throat, fever, mouth sores, easy bruising, nosebleed, purplish spots on skin, skin rash, hives, swelling around the face, difficult breathing, wheezing, tightness in the chest, slow heartbeat, fatigue, extreme sleepiness during the day, yellowish discoloration of the skin and eyes, depression, slurred speech, confusion, headache, unsteadiness, unusual nervousness or excitement, nightmares, hallucinations, anxiety, delirium, impaired vision, sleeplessness

Effects of Long-Term Use: anemia, dependence

Habit-Forming Possibility: This drug can lead to both physical and psychological dependence. This drug has potential for abuse since tolerance to it can develop easily.

Precautions and Suggestions:

Foods and beverages:
* No restrictions on foods.
* Avoid alcoholic beverages.

Other medicines, prescription and nonprescription:
* Phenobarbital may interact with anticonvulsants, central nervous system depressants (sedatives, sleeping aids, antihistamines, tranquilizers, phenothiazines, alcohol), antidepressants, antibiotics (tetracycline, doxycycline, chloramphenicol), anticoagulants, digitoxin, quinidine, furosemide, antidiabetic drugs, isoniazid, the antifungal griseofulvin, sulfa drugs, steroid drugs, oral contraceptives, theophylline, and aminophylline.
* Some of the forms of phenobarbital contain a dye called *tartrazine*, which may cause allergic-type reactions (including bronchial asthma) in some people, especially those sensitive to aspirin.

Other:
* If this drug causes you to become drowsy, do not engage in activities that require alertness, such as driving a car or operating potentially dangerous machinery.

- Do not change the prescribed dosage without consulting your doctor.
- Do not stop taking this drug suddenly; if you have been taking phenobarbital for an extended period of time, the drug must be stopped gradually.
- In older persons, phenobarbital may cause a reduction in the body temperature (hypothermia). During cold weather, dress warmly and ask your doctor to prescribe the minimum dosage.
- Never forget that this drug can be habit-forming.

Medical Tests:

- Your doctor may want to conduct tests to monitor the therapy.
- Phenobarbital may affect the results of some blood and urine tests.
- Any drug may affect the results and accuracy of a medical test. If a doctor recommends a medical or laboratory test for any condition, inform the doctor that you are taking this drug.

POTASSIUM CHLORIDE REPLACEMENT (GENERIC)

Ingredient(s): potassium chloride

Equivalent Product(s): Cena-K, Kaochlor, Kaon-Cl, Kato, Kay Ciel, Keff, K-Lor, Klor-Con, Klor-10%, Klorvess, Klotrix, K-Lyte/Cl, Kolyum, K-Tab, Micro-K, Pfiklor, Potachlor, Potage, Potasalan, Potassine, Rum-K, SK-Potassium Chloride, Slow-K

Used for: treatment or prevention of potassium deficiency caused by diuretics, dehydration, dietary lack, or surgery

Dosage Form and Strength: liquid, powder, effervescent tablets, tablets, enteric-coated tablets, sustained-release capsules, all available in various strengths

Storage: Store in tightly closed containers away from light.

Before Using This Drug, Tell Your Doctor: if you have any stomach or intestinal problems, including ulcers or blockages; Addison's disease; heart disease; kidney disease; urination difficulties; dehydration; heat cramps; diabetes; severe burns; adrenal gland insufficiency; high blood levels of potassium; or a certain type of muscle spasm (myotonia congenita). Tell your doctor about any drugs, prescription or nonprescription, you are taking and about any allergies you have or any family history of allergies.

This Drug Should Not Be Used If: you have kidney disease, untreated Addison's disease, high levels of potassium in your body, acute dehydration, heat cramps, myotonia congenita, or an allergy to potassium chloride supplements. This drug should not be used if you are taking potassium-sparing diuretics (spironolactone, triamterene, or amiloride) or aldosterone-inhibiting agents. The solid dosage forms should not be used by those who have an intestinal condition that would delay the passage of the drug though the gastrointestinal tract (this could include chronic constipation).

How to Use: Take this drug with food or immediately after a meal to prevent stomach upset. Measure the liquid form with a medical teaspoon; an ordinary kitchen teaspoon is not accurate enough. Dilute each dose of the liquid, powder, or effervescent tablet in four ounces of cold water or juice (do not use tomato juice unless your doctor orders it; it contains a great deal of sodium). Wait for the medication to be dissolved completely and to stop fizzing before drinking it. Sip it slowly. The tablets and capsules should be swallowed whole.

Time Required for Drug to Take Effect: 12 to 24 hours

Missing a Dose: Take the missed dose as soon as you remember, unless it is within two hours of the next dose. In that case, do not take the missed dose, but return to your regular dosing schedule. Do not double the next dose.

Symptoms of Overdose: weakness, listlessness, mental confusion, weakness and heaviness of the legs, muscle weakness, numbness or tingling, low blood pressure, heartbeat irregularities, changes in heart function, heart arrest, convulsions

Side Effects:

Minor and expected:
- nausea, vomiting, diarrhea, abdominal discomfort

Serious adverse reactions (CALL YOUR DOCTOR):
- black, tarry stools; vomiting blood; confusion; anxiety; numbness or tingling; weakness; weakness and heaviness of the legs; irregular heartbeat; difficult breathing; severe stomach pain

Effects of Long-Term Use: possible development of anemia in some individuals

Habit-Forming Possibility: none

Precautions and Suggestions:

Foods and beverages:
- No restrictions on beverages.
- Consult your doctor before using a salt substitute; salt substitutes often contain large amounts of potassium, which could lead to an overdose of potassium in your body.
- Avoid eating large quantities of foods rich in potassium.

Other medicines, prescription and nonprescription:
- Potassium taken with potassium-sparing diuretics such as triamterene, spironolactone, or amiloride can lead to dangerously high levels of potassium in the body.
- Potassium also may interact with digitalis and aldosterone antagonists.

Other:
- Some potassium chloride supplements contain a dye called *tartrazine* that may cause an allergic reaction in susceptible persons, many of whom are sensitive or allergic to aspirin.
- Do not increase your dose or take it longer than prescribed unless instructed to do so by your doctor.
- If you experience any of the minor side effects listed above, you may be able to eliminate them by diluting each dose with more water or juice.

Medical Tests:

- Your doctor may want to conduct periodic blood tests to monitor the blood levels of potassium and hemoglobin (to detect anemia).
- Your doctor may also perform periodic electrocardiograms to watch for any changes in the heart.
- Any drug may affect the results and accuracy of a medical test. If a doctor recommends a medical or laboratory test for any condition, inform the doctor that you are taking this drug.

PREDNISONE (GENERIC)

Ingredient(s): prednisone

Equivalent Product(s): Cortan, Deltasone, Fernisone, Liqui Pred, Meticorten, Orasone, Panasol, Prednicen-M, SK-Prednisone, Sterapred

Used for: treatment of inflammation caused by allergies or diseases, including asthma. It is also used to treat disorders of the glandular (endocrine) system.

Dosage Form and Strength: tablets—1 mg, 2.5 mg, 5 mg, 19 mg, 20 mg, 25 mg, 50 mg; syrup—5 mg per 5 ml

Storage: Store away from light in a tightly closed container.

Before Using This Drug, Tell Your Doctor: if you have a history of liver or kidney disease; ulcer or stomach problems; Cushing's syndrome; myasthenia gravis; tuberculosis; bone disease; diabetes; seizures; blood or heart disorders; high blood pressure; cataract; osteoporosis; glaucoma; cirrhosis; any infection, especially fungal and also chicken pox or shingles; herpes simplex infection in the eyes; or an underactive thyroid gland. Also, tell your doctor about any drugs, prescription or nonprescription, you are using (especially aspirin; diabetes medicine, including insulin; anticonvulsants; and antibiotics) and about any allergies you have or any family history of allergies.

This Drug Should Not Be Used If: you have an allergy to its ingredient, a bodywide fungal infection, an active herpes simplex eye infection, or active tuberculosis or if you have recently received an immunization or vaccination.

How to Use: Take this drug with food or milk. If you are taking a single dose each day or each alternate day, take the dose before 9:00 A.M. Multiple daily doses should be taken at evenly spaced intervals throughout the day. Do not stop taking this drug without talking to your doctor.

Time Required for Drug to Take Effect: Benefits may be apparent in 24 to 48 hours. The dosage may then have to be adjusted to provide maximum benefit; this usually occurs in four to 10 days. If you are taking prednisone on a long-term basis, it is important to adjust the dosage so that the smallest possible dose that will still achieve the necessary effect is given.

Missing a Dose: If you are taking a dose once a day, take the missed dose as soon as you remember. If you do not remember until the next day, do not take the missed dose at all, but follow your regular schedule. If you are taking prednisone every other day, take the missed dose as soon as you remember. If you miss the scheduled time by an entire day, go ahead and take the dose, but then skip a day before resuming the regular schedule. Do not double the dose. If you are taking prednisone more than once a day, take the missed dose as soon as possible and return to the regular schedule. If it is time or almost time for the next dose, double the dose. If you miss more than one dose, call your doctor for instructions.

Symptoms of Overdose: fluid retention, swelling of hands and feet, confusion, anxiety, depression, nervousness, stomach cramping or pain, flushed face, changes in behavior, severe headache, convulsions

Side Effects:

Minor and expected:
- nervousness, restlessness, sleeping problems, indigestion, increased susceptibility to bruising and to infections, weight gain, increased sweating, dizziness

Serious adverse reactions (CALL YOUR DOCTOR):
- blurred vision; increased thirst; frequent urination; skin rash; thin skin; purplish discoloration of skin; dark patches on skin; unusual bruising; convulsions; headache; mood changes; slow healing of wounds; sores in the mouth; muscle weakness or pain; bloody or black, tarry stools; nausea; vomiting; severe indigestion; unusual fatigue; menstrual irregularities; swelling of legs, feet, or face; increased hair growth; unexplained fever or sore throat; irregular heartbeat; emotional disturbances

Effects of Long-Term Use: weight gain, thinning of skin, loss of bone strength resulting in possible fractures, increase in blood sugar (possibly leading to diabetes), eye problems

Habit-Forming Possibility: Long-term use may lead to functional dependence in which a body function becomes dependent on the drug to do the job of the function. If the drug is withdrawn suddenly, that body function is not able to reestablish itself.

Precautions and Suggestions:

Foods and beverages:
- During long-term use, a high-protein diet is recommended.
- Ask your doctor if you should also eat more potassium-rich foods.

Other medicines, prescription and nonprescription:
- Prednisone interacts with aspirin, phenobarbital, tuberculosis drugs, ephedrine, phenytoin, some antibiotics, anticoagulants, diuretics, digitalis, cholestyramine, colestipol, glaucoma medications, stimulants, indomethacin, antihistamines, chloral hydrate, glutethimide, phenylbutazone, propranolol, and oral contaceptics.

- This drug increases the need for insulin or oral antidiabetes medication in diabetics.
- There is a possibility that the effects of the bronchodilator theophylline may be increased if prednisone is given at the same time, but the evidence is not conclusive.
- Prednisone is a steroid drug and is powerful. Be certain to tell your doctor about any drugs or products, even something as common as aspirin, that you are taking when prednisone is prescribed.

Other:

- Do not stop taking this medicine suddenly. If prednisone is to be stopped, it must be done so in a gradual manner under careful medical supervision. If the use of this drug has caused functional dependence, stopping it abruptly does not give the body time to reestablish its functions.
- Do not take more than the prescribed dose, and be certain to follow your doctor's instructions carefully.
- Do not accept an immunization or vaccination while taking prednisone.
- If you are treated by any doctor or dentist, particularly if the treatment involves surgery, within a year of taking prednisone, tell the medical-care provider that you were or still are taking prednisone.
- If you use prednisone for an extended period of time, inform any care provider for up to two years after discontinuation that you used this drug in the past.
- If you are taking this drug for more than a short-term (one-week) treatment, you should wear or carry a medical identification notice that you are taking a steroid drug.
- You may require higher doses of prednisone during times of stress or illness.
- This drug may mask the signs of infection or allow infections to develop. Be alert to any sign of illness.
- If you reduce the dosage or withdraw from the drug, notify your doctor if you experience fatigue, loss of appetite, nausea, vomiting, diarrhea, weight loss, weakness, dizziness, or low blood sugar.

Medical Tests:

- Your doctor may want to check your blood pressure, weight, and vision at regular intervals while prednisone is being taken and perhaps for a month or two after the drug is discontinued.
- Other laboratory tests may be required to monitor your progress.

- Prednisone can affect the results of some thyroid, glucose, and cholesterol tests, as well as other laboratory tests.
- Any drug may affect the results and accuracy of a medical test. If a doctor recommends a medical or laboratory test for any condition, inform the doctor that you are taking this drug.

PREMARIN

Ingredient(s): conjugated estrogens

Equivalent Product(s): conjugated estrogens (generic), Estrocon, Evestrone

Used for: symptoms of menopause, treatment of some kinds of cancer, and possible prevention of osteoporosis. This drug is also used as an estrogen replacement for those women whose bodies do not produce enough estrogen naturally.

Dosage Form and Strength: tablets—0.3 mg, 0.625 mg, 0.9 mg, 1.25 mg, 2.5 mg

Storage: Store in a tightly closed container at room tempreature.

Before Using This Drug, Tell Your Doctor: if you have a history of cancer of the breast or reproductive system, diabetes, blood clot disorders, endometriosis, epilepsy, gallbladder disease, heart disease, high blood pressure, stroke, high blood levels of calcium, kidney disease, liver disease, depression, fibroid tumors of the uterus, abnormal vaginal bleeding, thyroid disorders, asthma, porphyria, or migraine headaches. Tell your doctor if you are a smoker. Tell your doctor about any drugs, prescription or nonprescription, you are taking and about any allergies you have or any family history of allergies.

This Drug Should Not Be Used If: you have blood clot disorders (or developed such disorders when using estrogen in the past), cancer of the breast or reproductive system, undiagnosed abnormal vaginal or genital bleeding, or an allergy to estrogens.

How to Use: Take Premarin with food to prevent stomach upset. Ask your doctor exactly when to take this drug; often doctors recommend that this drug be taken for three weeks with one week off each month.

Time Required for Drug to Take Effect: Consistent use for 10 to 20 days may be necessary to determine the effectiveness of this drug.

Missing a Dose: Take the missed dose as soon as you remember, unless it is almost time for the next dose. In that case, omit the missed dose and return to your regular dosing schedule. Do not double the next dose.

Symptoms of Overdose: nausea, vomiting, fluid retention, abnormal vaginal bleeding, breast discomfort

Side Effects:

Minor and expected:
- fluid retention, weight gain, breakthrough vaginal bleeding, enlarged and tender breasts, diarrhea, dizziness, headache, loss of appetite

Serious adverse reactions (CALL YOUR DOCTOR):
- difficult breathing, chest pain, lumps in breast, secretion from breast, eye pain, changes in vision, intolerance to contact lenses, depression, convulsions, changes in sexual desire, difficult urination, eye pain, severe and sudden headache, yellowish discoloration of skin and whites of eyes, breakthrough bleeding, changes in menstruation, vaginal discharge, nausea, vomiting, abdominal pain, changes in skin color, increased body hair, hives, pain in the calves of the leg or groin, weakness or numbness in arm or leg

Effects of Long-Term Use: increase in growth of uterine fibroid tumors; also, possible increased risk of cancer of the lining of the uterus

Habit-Forming Possibility: none

Precautions and Suggestions:

Foods and beverages:
- No restrictions.

Other medicines, prescription and nonprescription:
- The effects of estrogen can be decreased if it is taken with carbamazepine, ampicillin, phenobarbital, phenytoin, primidone, or rifampin.
- Premarin may also interact with anticoagulants, thyroid hormones, and some antidepressants.

Other:
- Do not smoke while taking Premarin. Smoking increases the risks of serious cardiovascular side effects from Premarin.

- Blood sugar tolerance may be decreased when estrogen is used; if you are a diabetic, monitor your blood glucose closely and consult your doctor about managing any changes or abnormalities.
- This drug can change your blood-clotting capability; be careful to avoid injuries.
- Premarin can cause you to become sensitive to sunlight, resulting in skin color changes. If you are exposed to the sun, wear protective clothing and use an effective sunscreen.
- Before any medical, surgical, or dental procedure, tell the health care provider that you are taking Premarin.
- Discuss with your doctor all the facts about estrogens and cancer.

Medical Tests:

- Your doctor will want to conduct periodic medical examinations, including a breast check and most definitely a Pap smear, a test to detect cancer of the cervix early. He or she may also want to perform periodic endometrial (lining of the uterus) screenings.
- Any drug may affect the results and accuracy of a medical test. If a doctor recommends a medical or laboratory test for any condition, inform the doctor that you are taking this drug.

PROCARDIA

Ingredient(s): nifedipine

Equivalent Product(s): none

Used for: treatment of various types of angina

Dosage Form and Strength: capsules— 10 mg

Storage: Store in tightly closed container at room temperature away from light and moisture.

Before Using This Drug, Tell Your Doctor: if you have heart disease, kidney disease, liver disease, gallbladder disease, or low blood pressure.

This Drug Should Not Be Used If: you are allergic to its ingredient.

How to Use: Take this drug with a full glass of water on an empty stomach one hour before or two hours after a meal, unless your doctor tells you to do otherwise. The capsule should be swallowed whole.

Time Required for Drug to Take Effect: begins within 20 minutes

Missing a Dose: Take the missed dose as soon as you remember, unless it is within two hours of the next dose. In that case, do not take the missed dose, but return to your regular dosing schedule. Do not double the next dose.

Symptoms of Overdose: slow heartbeat, low blood pressure

Side Effects:

Minor and expected:
- nervousness, sleep problems, blurred vision, headache, weakness, nausea, diarrhea, constipation, cramps, gas, abdominal discomfort

Serious adverse reactions (CALL YOUR DOCTOR):
- dizziness, light-headedness, fluid retention, heartbeat irregularities, fainting, rash, hives, fever, chills, sweating, shortness of breath, muscle cramps, joint stiffness or pain, sexual problems, flushing, chest pain, symptoms of a heart attack

Effects of Long-Term Use: possible effect on the gallbladder

Habit-Forming Possibility: none

Precautions and Suggestions:

Foods and beverages:
- No restrictions.

Other medicines, prescription and nonprescription:
- Procardia may interact with beta blockers (atenolol, metoprolol, nadolol, pindolol, propranolol, timolol), quinidine, digoxin, narcotic analgesics, quinine, anticonvulsants, nitroglycerin, and anticoagulants.

Other:
- If this drug makes you dizzy or gives you blurred vision, do not engage in activities that require alertness and sharp vision, such as driving a car or operating potentially dangerous machinery.
- Do not stop taking the medication abruptly. Ask your doctor how to stop taking the drug.
- Before any medical, surgical, or dental procedure, tell the health-care provider that you are taking Procardia.

Medical Tests:

- Your doctor may want to perform periodic tests to monitor your progress on this drug.
- Any drug may affect the results and accuracy of a medical test. If a doctor recommends a medical or laboratory test for any condition, inform the doctor that you are taking this drug.

PROVENTIL

Ingredient(s): albuterol

Equivalent Product(s): Ventolin

Used for: the relief of spasms in the airways of persons with reversible, obstructive airway conditions, such as asthma, bronchitis, or emphysema. It may also prevent exercise-induced bronchospasm.

Dosage Form and Strength: tablets—2 mg, 4 mg; inhaler—90 mcg (micrograms) per actuation

Storage: Store tablets in a dark, cool place. Store the inhaler away from heat or open flame. Do not puncture, break, or burn an inhaler.

Before Using This Drug, Tell Your Doctor: if you have any circulatory system problems, degenerative heart disease, high blood pressure, a history of seizures, overactive thyroid gland, enlarged prostate, or diabetes. Tell your doctor if you are using any other bronchodilators, including nonprescription, especially those containing epinephrine. Tell your doctor about any drugs, prescription or nonprescription, including digitalis, you are taking and about any allergies you have or any family history of allergies.

This Drug Should Not Be Used If: you have an allergy to the active ingredient in the drug or a history of circulatory system problems, particularly heartbeat irregularities.

How to Use: If stomach upset occurs, take the treatment along with food.

Time Required for Drug to Take Effect: tablets, within 30 minutes; inhaler, within 15 minutes

Missing a Dose: If you miss a dose by an hour or less, take it when you remember and return to the regular schedule for the next dose. If you miss a dose by more than an hour, wait until the next dose. Do not double the dose or exceed the recommended dosage for the entire day.

Symptoms of Overdose: pounding heart, irregular heartbeat, chest pain, fever, chills, cold sweats, paleness, nausea, vomiting, unusual dilation of the pupil of the eye, anxiety, tremors, convulsions, delirium, collapse

Side Effects:

Minor and expected:
- dry throat and mouth, nervousness, restlessness, sleeplessness, stomach upset, unusual taste in mouth

Serious adverse reactions (CALL YOUR DOCTOR):
- pounding heart, chest pain, heartbeat irregularities, dizziness, headache, trembling, flushing, persistent breathing difficulty, confusion, muscle cramps, vomiting, weakness, headache, drowsiness, chest pain

Effects of Long-Term Use: Tolerance to the drug may develop with prolonged use, but temporarily stopping the drug restores the drug's effectiveness. Discuss this with your doctor.

Habit-Forming Possibility: none known

Precautions and Suggestions:

Foods and beverages:
- No restrictions.

Other medicines, prescription and nonprescription:
- This drug may react with other bronchodilators, especially epinephrine; some antidepressants; some antihistamines; thyroid medicine; beta blockers; antihypertensive medications; diuretics; and some heart medicines.

Other:
- Take this drug only as instructed. Do not increase the dosage or take it more often than prescribed without consulting your doctor.
- If your symptoms do not improve or become worse while using this drug, call your doctor.
- Be certain you know how to use the inhaler. Ask your doctor and pharmacist for complete instructions.

Medical Tests:

- No known interference.
- Your doctor may perform laboratory tests to monitor your progress on this drug.
- Any drug may affect the results and accuracy of a medical test. If a doctor recommends a medical or laboratory test for any condition, inform the doctor that you are taking this drug.

SELDANE

Ingredient(s): terfenadine

Equivalent Product(s): none

Used for: relief of upper respiratory allergy symptoms. Its main advantage is that it does not cause as much drowsiness or have as strong a sedative effect as other antihistamines.

Dosage Form and Strength: tablets—60 mg

Storage: Store in tightly closed container at room temperature away from moisture and heat.

Before Using This Drug, Tell Your Doctor: if you have a history of lower respiratory disorders, including asthma, or liver disease. Tell your doctor about any drugs, prescription or nonprescription, you are taking and about any allergies you have or any family history of allergies.

This Drug Should Not Be Used If: you are allergic to its active ingredient (terfenadine) or inactive ingredients (cornstarch, gelatin, lactose, magnesium stearate, and sodium bicarbonate).

How to Use: Take this drug at the same time every day. Ask your doctor if you can take Seldane with food or milk to prevent stomach upset.

Time Required for Drug to Take Effect: begins within one-half hour, reaching a peak in two hours

Missing a Dose: Ask your doctor what to do if you miss a dose.

Symptoms of Overdose: possible low blood pressure and loss of consciousness. This drug is new (approved in late 1985 by the Food and Drug Administration), and therefore only one case of overdose has been observed. Thus, this description cannot be definitive at this point.

Side Effects:

Minor and expected:
- mild drowsiness, fatigue, increased appetite, dry mouth, nose, and throat

Serious adverse reactions (CALL YOUR DOCTOR):
- headache, dizziness, nervousness, weakness, abdominal discomfort, nausea, vomiting, sore throat, rash, loss of hair, breathing difficulty, depression, insomnia, menstrual disorders, muscle or joint

pain, nightmares, heartbeat irregularities, sweating, tingling or prickling sensations, tremor, urinary frequency, vision problems, yellowish discoloration of the skin

Effects of Long-Term Use: unknown at this time

Habit-Forming Possibility: none

Precautions and Suggestions:

Foods and beverages:
- No restrictions on food.
- Ask your doctor if you can drink alcoholic beverages while taking Seldane.

Other medicines, prescription and nonprescription:
- No interactions have been reported, but tell your doctor about any medication you take, either prescription or nonprescription, and ask if you can take Seldane at the same time.

Other:
- If Seldane causes you to feel even slightly drowsy or dizzy, do not engage in activities that require alertness, such as driving a car or operating potentially dangerous equipment.
- When Seldane first appeared on the market, several pharmacists, unfamiliar with this new drug, inadvertently filled the prescription with Feldene, a nonsteroidal anti-inflammatory. Be certain you understand the name and spelling of the drug being prescribed and convey that information to the pharmacist. Tell him or her that you are being treated for an allergy.
- Seldane is such a new drug that many facts about it may not have surfaced yet. If you have any questions about this drug, ask your doctor before you take the medication.

Medical Tests:

- Seldane may interfere with the results of some medical and laboratory tests. If a doctor recommends a medical or laboratory test for any condition, inform the doctor that you are taking this drug.

SYNTHROID

Ingredient(s): levothyroxine sodium

Equivalent Product(s): Levthroid, Noroxine

Used for: replacement of natural thyroid hormone that is not being produced because of a disorder or absence of the thyroid gland

Dosage Form and Strength: tablets—0.025 mg, 0.05 mg, 0.075 mg, 0.1 mg, 0.125 mg, 0.15 mg, 0.175 mg, 0.2 mg, 0.3 mg

Storage: Store in a tightly closed container at room temperature.

Before Using This Drug, Tell Your Doctor: if you have or have had angina; high blood pressure; a recent heart attack; heart disease; coronary artery disease; underactive adrenal, testicle, ovary, or pituitary glands; diabetes; or kidney disease. Tell your doctor about any drugs, prescription or nonprescription, you are taking and about any allergies you have or any family history of allergies.

This Drug Should Not Be Used If: you have excessive levels of thyroid hormone in your body, untreated Addison's disease, or an allergy to the drug's ingredient. If you have had a recent heart attack, angina, or high blood pressure, you should not take this drug unless you have an underactive thyroid gland that is complicating or influencing the heart condition.

How to Use: Take with a glass of water at the same time every day.

Time Required for Drug to Take Effect: varies, depending on the condition of the person taking the drug. You may be asked to take the drug on a consistent basis for two to three weeks and then be examined to determine if your dosage should be maintained or changed.

Missing a Dose: Take the missed dose as soon as you remember, unless it is almost time for the next dose. In that case, do not take the missed dose and return to your regular dosing schedule. Do not double the next dose. If you miss more than one dose, call your doctor.

Symptoms of Overdose: headache, irritability, nervousness, sweating, rapid heartbeat, increased movement in the intestine, menstrual irregularities

Side Effects:

Minor and expected:
- dry and puffy skin, constipation, drowsiness, muscle aches, lack of energy, weight gain

Serious adverse reactions (CALL YOUR DOCTOR):
- pounding heart, rapid heartbeat, heartbeat irregularities, chest pain, headache, tremor, nervousness, nausea, insomnia, abdominal cramps, change in appetite, diarrhea, skin rash, weight loss,

sweating, menstrual irregularities, intolerance to heat, fever, irritability, nervousness, increased movement in the intestine

Effects of Long-Term Use: This drug is usually intended to be used on a long-term basis, often for life.

Habit-Forming Possibility: none

Precautions and Suggestions:

Foods and beverages:
* No restrictions.

Other medicines, prescription and nonprescription:
* Synthroid may change the dosage requirements of insulin and oral antidiabetic drugs.
* Estrogen also may change the dosage requirements for Synthroid.
* Synthroid may increase the effects of anticoagulants and possibly lead to bleeding problems.
* Epinephrine may interact with Synthroid in persons with heart disease.
* Cholestyramine may impair the body's absorption of Synthroid.
* Synthroid also may interact with heart drugs (such as digitalis), phenobarbital, phenytoin, some antidepressants, and some nonprescription preparations for coughs, colds, allergy, sinus, or weight loss.

Other:
* You may be required to take this medication for life if you have an underactive thyroid gland.
* Do not change brands of this drug without consulting your doctor.
* Some forms of this drug contain a dye called *tartrazine* that can cause an allergic reaction in susceptible persons (often those with a sensitivity to aspirin).
* Recently, because of the development of improved measuring processes, some thyroid medications were found to contain less of the hormone than they were labeled to contain. Manufacturers corrected this, which means that the dose you take may now be larger than needed. Discuss your dosage needs with your doctor.

Medical Tests:

* Synthroid may affect the results of some laboratory tests.
* Other drugs may affect the results of thyroid function tests, which your doctor may want to perform on a periodic basis to monitor your progress. Be certain to tell any doctor or health-care provider that you are taking Synthroid before any laboratory or medical tests.

TAGAMET

Ingredient(s): cimetidine

Equivalent Product(s): none

Used for: treatment and prevention of duodenal and gastric ulcers; also used to treat hypersecretory conditions, such as Zollinger-Ellison syndrome, systemic mastocytosis, and multiple endocrine adenomas

Dosage Form and Strength: tablets—200 mg, 300 mg, 400 mg; liquid—300 mg per 5 ml; twice-a-day regimen—400 mg

Storage: Store in tightly closed container at room temperature away from light. Do not freeze.

Before Using This Drug, Tell Your Doctor: if you have a low sperm count, kidney disease, organic brain syndrome, liver disease, arthritis, or any severe illnesses. Tell your doctor about any drugs, prescription or nonprescription, you are taking and about any allergies you have or any family history of allergies.

This Drug Should Not Be Used If: you are allergic to its ingredient.

How to Use: Take Tagamet with food or immediately after meals. Do not crush or chew the tablets; they have an unpleasant taste and odor. If you are using the liquid form, measure your dose with a medical teaspoon; an ordinary kitchen teaspoon is not accurate enough. Do not take an antacid at the same time as you take your dose.

Time Required for Drug to Take Effect: The drug's action begins in one hour and reaches a peak in one and one-half to two hours. Your doctor may want you to take this drug for six weeks on a consistent schedule to allow time for an ulcer to heal.

Missing a Dose: Take the missed dose as soon as you remember, unless it is almost time for the next dose. In that case, do not take the missed dose, but return to your regular dosing schedule. Do not double the next dose.

Symptoms of Overdose: rapid heartbeat, difficult breathing (in animal studies only), possible confusion or slurred speech in susceptible persons

Side Effects:

Minor and expected:
- drowsiness, dizziness, diarrhea, headache, muscle pain

Serious adverse reactions (CALL YOUR DOCTOR):
- joint pain, impotence, breast enlargement in men and women, unexplained sore throat and fever, hallucinations, confusion, delirium, speech difficulties, loss of coordination, double vision, heartbeat irregularities, yellowish discoloration of the skin and whites of eyes, skin loss, loss of hair, unusual bleeding or bruising

Effects of Long-Term Use: effect on the liver (reversible), possible breast enlargement; prolonged use should be avoided, if possible

Habit-Forming Possibility: none

Precautions and Suggestions:

Foods and beverages:
- Follow the diet recommended by your doctor. He or she may restrict certain foods to promote healing and recovery.
- Your doctor may restrict your intake of caffeine-containing beverages—coffee, tea, colas, cocoa—to reduce the possibility of increase in stomach acid.
- Ask your doctor before you drink alcoholic beverages.

Other medicines, prescription and nonprescription:
- Cigarette smoking reverses the effective action of this drug on secretion of stomach acid.
- The risk of developing blood disorders increases if Tagamet is taken along with anticancer drugs.
- Tagamet may decrease the blood levels of digoxin and therefore the effectiveness of digoxin.
- Tagamet decreases the absorption of ketoconazole; at least two hours should elapse between doses.
- The effects of carbamazepine may be increased if taken with Tagamet.
- Antacids may inhibit the absorption of Tagamet; therefore, antacids should be taken between doses of Tagamet.
- Tagamet also may interact with anticoagulants, phenytoin, beta blockers, lidocaine, theophylline and other respiratory drugs, morphine, metoclopramide, phenobarbital, chloramphenicol, and benzodiazepine tranquilizers (clorazepate, chlordiazepoxide, diazepam, flurazepam, halazepam, prazepam).

Other:
- If this drug makes you dizzy or drowsy, do not engage in activities that require alertness, such as driving a car or operating potentially dangerous equipment.

- Take Tagamet as long as your doctor recommends; do not stop taking it without consulting your doctor.
- Discuss with your doctor the advisability of taking over-the-counter drugs containing aspirin.

Medical Tests:

- Your doctor may want to perform periodic tests, including kidney and liver function tests, blood counts, and blood-clotting tests (if you take anticoagulants), to monitor your progress on this drug.
- Any drug may affect the results and accuracy of a medical test. If a doctor recommends a medical or laboratory test for any condition, inform the doctor that you are taking this drug.

TENORMIN

Ingredient(s): atenolol

Equivalent Product(s): none

Used for: treatment of high blood pressure

Dosage Form and Strength: tablets—50 mg, 100 mg

Storage: Store in a tightly closed container at room temperature away from light.

Before Using This Drug, Tell Your Doctor: if you have a history of heart disease; congestive heart failure; poor circulation in fingers and toes; asthma or any respiratory problems, including chronic obstructive pulmonary disease, bronchitis, and emphysema; hypoglycemia; diabetes; overactive thyroid gland; or kidney or liver disease. Tell your doctor about any drugs, prescription or nonprescription, you are taking and about any allergies you have or any family history of allergies.

This Drug Should Not Be Used If: you are allergic to its ingredient or have slow heartbeat, heart block greater than first degree, cardiogenic shock, or heart failure (unless it results from a condition treatable by this drug).

How to Use: This drug may be taken without regard to meals. Follow your doctor's advice about when to take this drug. Try to take the drug at the same time every day. Do not stop taking the drug abruptly unless your doctor instructs you to do so.

Time Required for Drug to Take Effect: one to two weeks

Missing a Dose: Take the missed dose as soon as you remember, unless you are due to take the next scheduled dose within eight hours if you take the drug once a day or within four hours if you take the drug more than once a day. In that case, omit the missed dose and maintain your regular schedule. Do not double the next dose.

Symptoms of Overdose: slow and/or weak pulse, weakness, dizziness on standing up, fainting, loss of consciousness, delirium, seizures, difficult or slowed breathing, bronchospasm, clammy skin

Side Effects:

Minor and expected:
- drowsiness, dry mouth, cold hands and feet, fatigue

Serious adverse reactions (CALL YOUR DOCTOR):
- sore throat, fever, light-headedness in upright position, breathing difficulties, night cough, wheezing, nasal stuffiness, chest pain, slow pulse (less than 60 beats per minute), retention of fluid, worsening of angina, heartbeat irregularities, dizziness, fainting, depression, lethargy, sleeplessness, anxiety, nervousness, nightmares or odd dreams, confusion, behavior changes, hallucinations, slurred speech, ringing in the ears, headache, short-term memory loss, numbness or tingling in fingers and toes, reduced sexual interest and/or ability, abdominal pain or cramping, nausea, vomiting, constipation, diarrhea, loss of appetite, urination difficulties and/or frequency, bruising, eye discomfort, dry and burning eyes, blurred vision, rash, itching, skin irritation, dry skin, sweating, changes in skin color, reversible baldness, joint pain, muscle cramps and pain

Effects of Long-Term Use: Long-term use in high doses may lead to reduced strength of heart muscle, which may increase the risk of heart failure.

Habit-Forming Possibility: none

Precautions and Suggestions:

Foods and beverages:
- No food restrictions.
- Consult your doctor before drinking alcoholic beverages because alcohol may increase the action of Tenormin.

Other medicines, prescription and nonprescription:

- Tenormin may interact with anesthetics and should be discontinued gradually before any surgery. Be certain your doctor, surgeon, and/or dentist knows you are taking this drug before any surgical procedure is begun.
- Nicotine in tobacco may decrease the effectiveness of this drug. Ask your doctor about smoking while taking this drug.
- Tenormin may increase the effects of other high blood pressure medications, insulin and oral antidiabetic drugs, barbiturates, narcotics, and reserpine.
- Tenormin may decrease the effects of aspirin, cortisone, and other anti-inflammatory drugs. Tenormine also decreases the effects of antihistamines to treat allergies.
- Tenormin may also interact with digitalis, digoxin, verapamil, nifedipine, diltiazem, quinidine, phenytoin, chlorpromazine, monoamine oxidase inhibitors, phenothiazines, cimetidine, oral contraceptives, furosemide, hydralazine, rifampin, phenobarbital, indomethacin, prazosin, isoproterenol, norepinephrine, dopamine, dobutamine, theophylline and other bronchodilators, and clonidine.

Other:

- Do not stop taking this drug abruptly unless your doctor instructs you to do so; this drug must be discontinued gradually.
- If this drug makes you dizzy or drowsy, do not engage in activities that require alertness, such as driving a car or operating potentially dangerous machinery.
- This drug may hide the signs of impending hypoglycemia and change blood sugar levels in diabetics. If you are a diabetic, work with your doctor to adjust your diabetes medications to compensate for this drug.
- Do not take any nonprescription preparations for cough, cold, allergy, or sinus problems without calling your doctor.

Medical Tests:

- This drug may interfere with glucose and insulin tolerance tests.
- If you are taking Tenormin on a long-term basis, your doctor may want to perform blood tests to monitor your progress.
- Your doctor may ask you to take your pulse each day; if it falls below 60 beats per minute, call your doctor.
- Your doctor will definitely want to check your blood pressure on a periodic basis.
- Any drug may affect the results and accuracy of a medical test. If a doctor recommends a medical or laboratory test for any condition, inform the doctor that you are taking this drug.

TETRACYCLINE (GENERIC)

Ingredient(s): tetracycline hydrochloride

Equivalent Product(s): Achromycin V, Cycline-250, Cyclopar, Delta-mycin, Nor-Tet, Panmycin, Retet, Robitet, SK-Tetracycline, Sumycin, Tetra-C, Tetracap, Tetracyn, Tetralan, Tetram

Used for: treatment of bacterial infections

Dosage Form and Strength: oral suspension—125 mg per 5 ml; capsules—100 mg, 250 mg, 500 mg; tablets—250 mg, 500 mg

Storage: Store in a cool, dark place.

Before Using This Drug, Tell Your Doctor: if you have diabetes, liver or kidney disease or a history of systemic lupus erythematosus, blood disorders, or aspirin sensitivity. Tell your doctor about any drugs, prescription or nonprescription, you are taking and about any allergies you have or any family history of allergies.

This Drug Should Not Be Used If: you are allergic to its ingredient.

How to Use: This drug should be taken on an empty stomach at least one hour before or two hours after a meal. Take the dose with a full glass of water. Do not take an antacid, a laxative, or any medication containing iron within three hours of a dose. Do not eat or drink any dairy products within two hours before or after taking a dose. Continue taking the medication for the full time prescribed by your doctor even if you seem well.

Time Required for Drug to Take Effect: varies, depending on the infection; usually two to five days

Missing a Dose: Take the missed dose immediately. If you do not remember until almost time for the next dose, take that next dose about halfway through the regular interval between doses. Then return to the normal schedule. Do not skip a dose or double the dose.

Symptoms of Overdose: possible nausea, vomiting, diarrhea

Side Effects:

Minor and expected:
- sensitivity to sunlight, loss of appetite, diarrhea, upset stomach, nausea, vomiting

Serious adverse reactions (CALL YOUR DOCTOR):
- dark-colored or swollen tongue, stomach pain, rash, hives, itching, difficulty in swallowing, sore throat, sores in mouth, hoarseness, headache, discolored nails, itching in genital and anal areas, fever, joint pain, difficulty in breathing

Effects of Long-Term Use: superinfection—that is, a second infection in addition to the infection being treated. A superinfection is caused by bacteria and other organisms that are not susceptible to or affected by the drug being used to treat the original infection. Thus, these organisms, which are normally too few in number to cause problems, grow unchecked and cause a second infection that may require treatment with a different drug.

Habit-Forming Possibility: none

Precautions and Suggestions:

Foods and beverages:
- Food and dairy products (milk and cheese) interfere with the absorption of tetracycline. Do not eat or drink dairy products within two hours before or after a dose.
- Avoid alcohol if you have a history of liver disease.

Other medicines, prescription and nonprescription:
- This drug interacts with penicillin, antacids, iron and mineral supplements, digoxin, anticoagulants, lithium, anticonvulsants, and theophylline (for asthma).
- This drug also interacts with some anesthetics. If you undergo any procedure that requires an anesthetic, be sure to tell the doctor or dentist that you are taking tetracycline.

Other:
- Do not use this drug beyond the expiration date and do not use it if it changes color or appearance. Outdated tetracycline can be poisonous.
- Some forms of this drug contain a dye called *tartrazine* that may cause an allergic reaction, especially in someone who is sensitive to aspirin.
- Don't expose yourself to sunlight without protective clothing and a sunscreen.

Medical Tests:

- In long-term therapy, your doctor may want to perform blood tests, liver and kidney function tests, and others to monitor your progress.
- Tetracycline can affect the results of some urine tests.
- Any drug may affect the results and accuracy of a medical test. If a doctor recommends a medical or laboratory test for any condition, inform the doctor that you are taking this drug.

THEOPHYLLINE (GENERIC)

Ingredient(s): theophylline

Equivalent Product(s): Accurbron, Aerolate, Aquaphyllin, Asmalix, Bronkodyl, Constant-T, Duraphyl, Elixicon, Elixomin, Elixophyllin, LaBID, Lanophyllin, Liquophylline, Lixolin, Lodrane, Quibron-T Dividose, Respbid, Slo-bid, Slo-Phyllin, Somophyllin-T, Sustaire, Theo-24, Theobid, Theobron, Theoclear, Theo-Dur, Theolair, Theo-Lix, Theolixir, Theon, Theophyl, Theospan, Theostat, Theo-Time, Theovent, Uniphyl

Used for: treatment of breathing problems in asthma, chronic bronchitis, or emphysema

Dosage Form and Strength: capsules—50 mg, 100 mg, 200 mg, 250 mg; chewable tablets—100 mg; tablets—100 mg, 125 mg, 200 mg, 225 mg, 250 mg, 300 mg; elixir—80 mg, 112.5 mg, both per 15 ml; solution—80 mg per 15 ml; liquid—80 mg, 150 mg, 160 mg, all per 15 ml; syrup—80 mg, 150 mg, both per 15 ml; suspension—300 mg per 15 ml; timed-release capsules—50 mg, 60 mg, 65 mg, 75 mg, 100 mg, 125 mg, 130 mg, 200 mg, 250 mg, 260 mg, 300 mg, 400 mg, 500 mg

Storage: Store in a dry, tightly covered container.

Before Using This Drug, Tell Your Doctor: if you have any form of heart, blood, respiratory, liver, or kidney disease; high blood pressure; overactive thyroid gland; a history of congestive heart failure, cor pulmonale, or alcoholism; enlarged prostate; inflammation of the stomach or an ulcer; or a sensitivity to caffeine. Also, tell your doctor about any drugs, prescription or nonprescription, you are taking and about any allergies you have or any family history of allergies.

This Drug Should Not Be Used If: you are allergic to this drug or any similar drugs, if you have an ulcer or other stomach inflammation, or if you are sensitive to caffeine. This drug should be used with caution by persons over 50 years of age, especially men.

How to Use: Theophylline is more effective if taken on an empty stomach; however, if stomach upset occurs, ask your doctor if you can take it with food. If possible, take with a full glass of water one hour before or two hours after a meal. Take every six hours around the clock, except for timed-release capsules. Do not crush or chew coated or timed-release forms.

Time Required for Drug to Take Effect: The effect begins in 15 to 30 minutes and reaches a maximum benefit in 1 to 2 hours. Depending on the dosage form and strength, the drug's benefit begins to subside in six to ten hours.

Missing a Dose: If you remember the missed dose within an hour of its normally scheduled time, take the missed dose. Then return to your normal schedule. If more than an hour has passed since the normally scheduled time, wait until the next regular dose. Do not double the dose. Ask your doctor about what to do for your individual situation if you miss a dose.

Symptoms of Overdose: loss of appetite, nausea, restlessness, irritability, irregular heartbeat, occasional vomiting, headache, confusion. Some people may display restlessness and hyperactivity that may lead to convulsions and death without warning symptoms of poisoning.

Side Effects:

Minor and expected:
- nervousness, insomnia

Serious adverse reactions (CALL YOUR DOCTOR):
- vomiting, skin rash or hives, irregular heartbeat, stomach pain, rapid breathing, severe depression, abnormal behavior (withdrawal alternating with hyperactivity), headache, confusion, restlessness, nausea, diarrhea, dizziness, changes in speech, difficult urination, loss of appetite, irritability, convulsions, breathing difficulty, loss of body fluids, thirst, fever

Effects of Long-Term Use: stomach irritation

Habit-Forming Possibility: none

Precautions and Suggestions:

Foods and beverages:
- Avoid charcoal-broiled food and a high-protein/low-carbohydrate diet. Try to balance your diet between high-protien/low-carbohydrate and low-protein/high-carbohydrate, either of which can affect the way the body uses and eliminates theophylline. The diet should remain as constant as possible. Do not eat or drink large amounts of anything containing caffeine or chocolate (don't forget that many colas contain caffeine).
- Ask your doctor for suggestions about the most beneficial diet.

Other medicines, prescription and nonprescription:
- Theophylline interacts with other drugs for asthma, including ephedrine (used in some nasal decongestants); phenobarbital; some antibiotics (erythromycin, troleandomycin, clindamycin); the ulcer medication cimetidine; some antacids; and the anticonvulsant Dilantin.
- Theophylline may interact with the worm medicine called *thiabendazole*.
- Theophylline may interact with gout medicines (allopurinal, probenecid, sulfinpyrazone), lithium, reserpine, furosemide, anticoagulants, digitalis, muscle relaxants, beta blockers, and antacids.
- If your doctor recommends a flu vaccination for you, remind the doctor that you are taking theophylline, which can interact with a flu vaccination.
- Theophylline can interact with some anesthetics; if you face any procedure that requires anesthesia, be sure to tell the doctor or dentist that you are taking theophylline.
- Always consult your doctor before taking any other medicines, including over-the-counter products.

Other:
- If you smoke tobacco or marijuana, tell your doctor of your smoking habits. Smoking can affect the action of this drug.

Medical Tests:

- This drug may affect the results of some urine tests and of tests for uric acid levels.
- Usage is monitored by measuring blood levels; short-acting theophylline is monitored two hours after the dose is given, and the long-acting form is measured four hours after the dose is given. This test can be affected by concurrent use of furosemide, phenylbutazone, probenecid, theobromine, coffee, tea, cola, chocolate, and acetaminophen.

• Any drug may affect the results and accuracy of a medical test. If a doctor recommends a medical or laboratory test for any condition, inform the doctor that you are taking this drug.

TIMOPTIC

Ingredient(s): timolol maleate

Equivalent Product(s): none

Used for: treatment of glaucoma

Dosage Form and Strength: solution—0.25%, 0.5%

Storage: Store in a tightly closed container at room temperature away from light. Do not refrigerate or freeze. If the solution changes color, discard it; a change of color indicates loss of strength.

Before Using This Drug, Tell Your Doctor: if you have asthma, including bronchial asthma or chronic obstructive pulmonary disease; heart failure; slow heartbeat; heart block greater than first degree; myasthenia gravis; or diabetes. Tell your doctor about any drugs, prescription or nonprescription, you are taking, especially beta blockers, and about any allergies you have or any family history of allergies.

This Drug Should Not Be Used If: you are allergic to its ingredient or if you have asthma, bronchial asthma, severe chronic obstructive pulmonary disease, or uncontrolled heart failure. This drug should be used with caution by persons with heart disease or diabetes.

How to Use: Wash your hands before applying the medication. Tilt your head back and make a pouch below the eye by pulling down the lower eyelid with one hand. Without allowing the dropper to touch the eye or eyelid, place the prescribed amount of solution in the pouch and, while keeping eye open, apply gentle pressure to the bridge of the nose at the inside corner of the eye for about one minute. This is done to prevent loss of medication into nose. Do not blink for at least 30 seconds. Do not rinse dropper, but simply replace it into the container. If you are using more than one kind of eyedrops, wait at least five minutes before applying the second kind of drops.

Time Required for Drug to Take Effect: The drug's action can begin in one half hour, reaching a peak in one to two hours, and the action may be maintained for as long as 24 hours. Your doctor may want to determine if this drug is effective for you after about four weeks of consistent use.

Missing a Dose: Apply the missed dose as soon as you remember, unless it is almost time for the next dose. In that case, omit the missed dose and return to your regular dosing schedule. Even if you only use the medication once a day and you don't remember until the next day, skip the missed dose. Do not double the next dose.

Symptoms of Overdose: disturbance in vision, possible slowing of heartbeat and lowering of blood pressure

Side Effects:

Minor and expected:
- stinging or eye irritation at time of application

Serious adverse reactions (CALL YOUR DOCTOR):
- persistent stinging or irritation that lasts more than a few minutes after application. If this drug is used correctly, major side effects are rare. However, there have been rare occurrences of serious adverse reactions in some individuals, including changes in vision, slow heartbeat, lowered blood pressure, fainting, bronchospasm, breathing difficulty, heart failure, hidden lowered blood sugar in diabetics, rash, hives, headache, dry mouth, loss of appetite, indigestion, nausea, dizziness, possible impotence, fatigue, confusion, hallucinations, depression, anxiety, sleepiness, palpitations, or discoloration of fingernails and toenails.

Effects of Long-Term Use: possible development of tolerance to the drug

Habit-Forming Possibility: none

Precautions and Suggestions:

Foods and beverages:
- No restrictions.

Other medicines, prescription and nonprescription:
- Timoptic may interact with other beta blockers.

Other:
- If this drug affects your ability to see clearly, do not drive a car or operate potentially dangerous equipment.
- Before any surgery or dental procedure, tell the health-care provider that you are using this drug.
- Do not use other eye medications, including nonprescription preparations, unless instructed to do so by your doctor.
- Do not use more of this medication, or use it more often, than your doctor prescribes.

Medical Tests:

- Your doctor will want to check your internal eye pressure (the glaucoma test) on a periodic basis while you are using this drug.
- Any drug may affect the results and accuracy of a medical test. If a doctor recommends a medical or laboratory test for any condition, inform the doctor that you are taking this drug.

TRANXENE

Ingredient(s): clorazepate dipotassium

Equivalent Product(s): none

Used for: treatment of anxiety, certain types of seizures, and alcohol withdrawal

Dosage Form and Strength: capsules—3.75 mg, 7.5 mg, 15 mg; tablets—3.75 mg, 7.5 mg, 15 mg; tablets, single-dose—11.25 mg (called Tranxene-SD Half Strength), 22.5 mg (called Tranxene-SD)

Storage: Store in tightly closed container at room temperature away from light.

Before Using This Drug, Tell Your Doctor: if you have a history of drug dependence, mental illness, depression, acute narrow-angle glaucoma, epilepsy, liver or kidney disease, Parkinson's disease, myasthenia gravis, or lung disease. Tell your doctor about any drugs, prescription or nonprescription, you are taking and about any allergies you have or any family history of allergies.

This Drug Should Not Be Used If: you have a psychotic illness, acute narrow-angle glaucoma, or an allergy to its ingredient or to similar drugs.

How to Use: Take this drug with a glass of water or with food to prevent stomach upset. Do not crush or chew Tranxene-SD. Do not use antacids at the same time, because they may inhibit the absorption of Tranxene.

Time Required for Drug to Take Effect: one to two hours

Missing a Dose: Take the missed dose as soon as you remember, unless more than an hour has passed. In that case, omit the missed dose and return to your regular dosing schedule. Do not double the next dose.

Symptoms of Overdose: extreme drowsiness, confusion, lethargy, loss of coordination, loss of muscle tone, loss of consciousness

Side Effects:

Minor and expected:
- mild drowsiness, lethargy, unsteadiness

Serious adverse reactions (CALL YOUR DOCTOR):
- sleepiness, depression, apathy, fatigue, light-headedness, disorientation, confusion, restlessness, crying, delirium, headache, slurred speech, fainting, rigidity and tremor, loss of muscle tone, dizziness, nervousness, exaggerated sense of well-being, irritability, difficulty in concentrating, weakness, vivid dreams, excitement, anxiety, hallucinations, muscle spasms, insomnia, sleep problems, anger, constipation, diarrhea, dry mouth, nausea, vomiting, loss of or change in appetite, difficulty in swallowing, stomach problems, incontinence, changes in sexual desire, difficulty in urinating, menstrual irregularities, heartbeat irregularities, changes in blood pressure, palpitations, fluid retention, vision problems, hearing problems, nasal stuffiness, rash, hives, itching, hiccoughs, fever, sweating, prickling or tingling sensations, enlarged breasts in men and women, breathing problems, yellowish discoloration of skin and whites of eyes, gain or loss of weight, joint pain

Effects of Long-Term Use: possible physical or psychological dependence, impairment of blood cell formation and of liver function

Habit-Forming Possibility: Tranxene can lead to physical and/or psychological dependence if taken in large doses for a long period of time.

Precautions and Suggestions:

Foods and beverages:
- No food restrictions, but large amounts of caffeine (coffee, tea, colas, chocolate) can reduce the calming action of this drug.
- Avoid alcohol.

Other medicines, prescription and nonprescription:
- The action of Traxene is increased by phenothiazine tranquilizers, antihistamines, narcotics, barbiturates, monoamine oxidase inhibitors, tricyclic antidepressants, anticonvulsants, muscle relaxants, and painkillers.
- Tranxene also may interact with rifampin, levodopa, disulfiram, isoniazid, cimetidine, and anticoagulants.
- Cigarette smoking may interfere with the effects of Tranxene.
- Antacids may interfere with the absorption of this drug.

Other:

- Do not engage in activities that require alertness, such as driving a car or operating potentially dangerous equipment.
- Do not increase the dosage without consulting your doctor.
- Do not stop taking this drug abruptly; it must be discontinued gradually.
- Do not take any nonprescription preparations for cough, cold, allergy, weight loss, or sinus problems without consulting your doctor.

Medical Tests:

- Tranxene may interfere with the results of some medical tests.
- Your doctor may want to conduct blood cell counts and liver function tests to monitor your progress on this drug.
- Any drug may affect the results and accuracy of a medical test. If a doctor recommends a medical or laboratory test for any condition, inform the doctor that you are taking this drug.

TYLENOL WITH CODEINE

Ingredient(s): acetaminophen and codeine

Equivalent Product(s): Aceta with Codeine, acetaminophen with codeine (generic), Anacin-3 with Codeine No. 3 and No. 4, Bayapap with Codeine, Capital with Codeine, Empracet with Codeine No. 3 and No. 4, Panadol with Codeine No. 3 and No. 4, SK-APAP with Codeine, Ty-Tab #3 and #4

Used for: relief of mild to severe pain

Dosage Form and Strength: tablets—7.5 mg codeine and 300 mg acetaminophen (No. 1), 15 mg codeine and 300 mg acetaminophen (No. 2), 30 mg codeine and 300 mg acetaminophen (No. 3), 60 mg codeine and 300 mg acetaminophen (No. 4); elixir—12 mg codeine and 120 mg acetaminophen

Storage: All dosage forms should be stored at room temperature. Do not freeze.

Before Using This Drug, Tell Your Doctor: if you have liver or kidney disease, asthma or other respiratory conditions, blood disorders, brain disease, head injuries, epilepsy, acute abdominal problems, colitis, gallbladder disease or stones, heart disease, lung disease, thyroid disease, prostate problems, narrowing of the urethra, or mental illness. Tell your doctor if you have a history of drug dependence, alcoholism, delirum tremens, cerebral arteriosclerosis, Addison's disease, curvature of the spine (kyphoscoliosis), or severe central nervous system depression. Tell your doctor about any drugs, prescription or nonprescription, you are taking and about any allergies you have or any family history of allergies.

This Drug Should Not Be Used· If: you are allergic to either of its ingredients. This drug is not recommended for use during a bout of diarrhea caused by poisoning until the poison is eliminated from the body.

How to Use: Take this drug with water or food. For the most effective action, take the drug at the onset of pain rather than waiting until the pain becomes severe. If you are using the elixir, measure the dose in a medical teaspoon; an ordinary kitchen teaspoon is not accurate enough.

Time Required for Drug to Take Effect: 15 to 30 minutes

Missing a Dose: Take the missed dose as soon as you remember, unless it is almost time for the next dose. In that case, omit the missed dose and return to your regular dosing schedule. Do not double the next dose.

Symptoms of Overdose: severe drowsiness, nausea, vomiting, restlessness, excitability, deep sleep, convulsions, clammy skin, shallow breathing, constricted pupils, limpness, abdominal pain, yellowish discoloration of skin and whites of eyes

Side Effects:

Minor and expected:
- drowsiness, dry mouth, constipation, light-headedness

Serious adverse reactions (CALL YOUR DOCTOR):
- rash, hives, itching, nausea, vomiting, dizziness, blurred vision, sweating, headache, sleeplessness, mood changes, tremors, uncoordinated muscles, difficulty in breathing, fear, anxiety, confusion, agitation, unexplained bruising or bleeding

Effects of Long-Term Use: possible physical and/or psychological dependence, as well as anemia

Habit-Forming Possibility: The codeine ingredient in this drug can lead to dependence when used in large doses and for a long period of time.

Precautions and Suggestions:

Foods and beverages:
- No food restrictions.
- Avoid alcoholic beverages and other medications containing alcohol as well as beverages containing caffeine.

Other medicines, prescription and nonprescription:
- This medication may interact with narcotics, sedatives, tranquilizers, anesthetics, barbiturates, antihistamines, painkillers, antidepressants, phenothiazines, and monoamine oxidase inhibitors.
- This drug may also interfere with aspirin, the antibiotic chloramphenicol, chlordiazepoxide, phenobarbital, oral contraceptives, or anticoagulants.
- There have been reports of reactions when narcotics such as codeine are taken at the same time as cimetidine (Tagamet), although no clear-cut cause-and-effect relationship has been established.

Other:
- If this drug makes you drowsy or dizzy, do not engage in activities that require alertness, such as driving a car or operating potentially dangerous machinery.

Medical Tests:

- This drug may interfere with some medical tests, especially liver tests.
- Your doctor may want to perform blood tests to monitor your progress on this drug.
- Any drug may affect the results and accuracy of a medical test. If a doctor recommends a medical or laboratory test for any condition, inform the doctor that you are taking this drug.

VALIUM

Ingredient(s): diazepam

Equivalent Product(s): diazepam (generic)

Used for: treatment of symptoms of anxiety, muscle spasms, alcohol withdrawal, and certain types of seizures

Dosage Form and Strength: tablets—2 mg, 5 mg, 10 mg

Storage: Store in a tightly closed container at room temperature away from light.

Before Using This Drug, Tell Your Doctor: if you have a history of drug dependence, mental illness, depression, acute narrow-angle glaucoma, epilepsy, liver or kidney disease, Parkinson's disease, myasthenia gravis, or lung disease. Tell your doctor about any drugs, prescription or nonprescription, you are taking and about any allergies you have or any family history of allergies.

This Drug Should Not Be Used If: you have a psychotic illness, acute narrow-angle glaucoma, or an allergy to its ingredient or to similar drugs.

How to Use: Take this drug with a glass of water or with food to prevent stomach upset. Do not use antacids at the same time, because they may inhibit absorption of Valium.

Time Required for Drug to Take Effect: one to two hours

Missing a Dose: Take the missed dose as soon as you remember, unless more than an hour has passed. In that case, omit the missed dose and return to your regular dosing schedule. Do not double the next dose.

Symptoms of Overdose: extreme drowsiness, confusion, lethargy, loss of coordination, loss of muscle tone, loss of consciousness

Side Effects:

Minor and expected:
- mild drowsiness, lethargy, unsteadiness

Serious adverse reactions (CALL YOUR DOCTOR):
- sleepiness, depression, apathy, fatigue, light-headedness, disorientation, confusion, restlessness, crying, delirium, headache, slurred speech, fainting, rigidity and tremor, loss of muscle tone, dizziness, nervousness, exaggerated sense of well-being, irritability, difficulty in concentrating, weakness, vivid dreams, excitement, anxiety, hallucinations, muscle spasms, insomnia, sleep problems, anger, constipation, nausea, vomiting, dry mouth, diarrhea, loss of or change in appetite, difficulty in swallowing, stomach problems, incontinence, changes in sexual desire, difficulty in urinating, menstrual irregularities, heartbeat irregularities, changes in blood pressure, palpitations, fluid retention, vision problems, hearing problems, nasal stuffiness, rash, hives, itching, hiccoughs, fever, sweating, prickling or tingling sensations, enlarged breasts in men and women, breathing problems, yellowish discoloration of skin and whites of eyes, gain or loss of weight, joint pain

Effects of Long-Term Use: possible physical or psychological dependence, impairment of blood cell formation and liver function

Habit-Forming Possibility: Valium can lead to physical and/or psychological dependence if taken in large doses for a long period of time

Precautions and Suggestions:

Foods and beverages:
- No food restrictions, but large amounts of caffeine (coffee, tea, colas, chocolate) can reduce the calming action of this drug.
- Avoid alcohol.

Other medicines, prescription and nonprescription:
- The action of Valium is increased by phenothiazine tranquilizers, antihistamines, narcotics, barbiturates, monoamine oxidase inhibitors, tricyclic antidepressants, anticonvulsants, muscle relaxants, and painkillers.
- Valium may also interact with rifampin, levodopa, disulfiram, isoniazid, valproic acid, oral contaceptives, cimetidine, and anticoagulants.
- Cigarette smoking may interfere with the effects of Valium.
- Antacids may interfere with the absorption of Valium.

Other:
- Do not engage in activities that require alertness, such as driving a car or operating potentially dangerous machinery.
- Do not increase the dosage without consulting with your doctor.
- Do not stop taking this drug abruptly; it must be discontinued gradually.
- Do not take any nonprescription preparations for cough, cold, allergy, weight loss, or sinus problems without consulting your doctor.

Medical Tests:

- Valium may interfere with the results of some medical tests.
- Your doctor may want to conduct blood cell counts and liver function tests to monitor your progress on this drug.
- Any drug may affect the results and accuracy of a medical test. If a doctor recommends a medical or laboratory test for any condition, inform the doctor that you are taking this drug.

XANAX

Ingredient(s): alprazolam

Equivalent Product(s): none

Used for: relief of anxiety, including anxiety associated with depression

Dosage Form and Strength: tablets—0.25 mg, 0.5 mg, 1 mg

Storage: Store in tightly closed container at room temperature away from light.

Before Using This Drug, Tell Your Doctor: if you have a history of drug dependence, mental illness, depression, acute narrow-angle glaucoma, epilepsy, liver or kidney disease, Parkinson's disease, myasthenia gravis, or lung disease. Tell the doctor about any drugs, prescription or nonprescription, you are taking and about any allergies you have or any family history of allergies.

This Drug Should Not Be Used If: you have a psychotic illness, acute narrow-angle glaucoma, or an allergy to Xanax's ingredient or to similar drugs.

How to Use: Take this drug with a glass of water or with food to prevent stomach upset. Ask your doctor if you can use antacids at the same time, because they may inhibit the absorption of Xanax.

Time Required for Drug to Take Effect: one to two hours

Missing a Dose: Take the missed dose as soon as you remember, unless more than an hour has passed. In that case, omit the missed dose and return to your regular dosing schedule. Do not double the next dose.

Symptoms of Overdose: extreme drowsiness, confusion, lethargy, loss of coordination, loss of muscle tone, loss of consciousness

Side Effects:

Minor and expected:
- mild drowsiness, lethargy, unsteadiness

Serious adverse reactions (CALL YOUR DOCTOR):
- sleepiness, depression, apathy, fatigue, light-headedness, disorientation, confusion, restlessness, crying, delirium, headache, slurred speech, fainting, rigidity and tremor, loss of muscle tone, dizziness, nervousness, exaggerated sense of well-being, irritability, difficulty in concentrating, weakness, vivid dreams, excitement, anxiety,

hallucinations, muscle spasms, insomnia, sleep problems, anger, constipation, diarrhea, dry mouth, nausea, vomiting, loss of or change in appetite, difficulty in swallowing, stomach problems, incontinence, changes in sexual desire, difficulty in urinating, menstrual irregularities, heartbeat irregularities, changes in blood pressure, palpitations, fluid retention, vision problems, hearing problems, nasal stuffiness, rash, hives, itching, hiccoughs, fever, sweating, prickling or tingling sensations, enlarged breasts in men and women, breathing problems, yellowish discoloration of skin and whites of eyes, gain or loss of weight, joint pain

Effects of Long-Term Use: possible physical or psychological dependence, impairment of blood cell formation and of liver function

Habit-Forming Possibility: Xanax can lead to physical and/or psychological dependence if taken in large doses for long periods of time.

Precautions and Suggestions:

Foods and beverages:
- No food restrictions, but large amounts of caffeine (coffee, tea, colas, chocolate) can reduce the calming action of this drug.
- Avoid alcohol.

Other medicines, prescription and nonprescription:
- The action of Xanax may be increased by phenothiazine tranquilizers, antihistamines, narcotics, barbiturates, monoamine oxidase inhibitors, tricyclic antidepressants, anticonvulsants, muscle relaxants, and painkillers.
- Xanax may also interact with rifampin, levodopa, disulfiram, isoniazid, cimetidine, and anticoagulants.
- Cigarette smoking may interfere with the effects of Xanax.

Other:
- Do not engage in activities that require alertness, such as driving a car or operating potentially dangerous machinery.
- Do not increase the dosage without consulting your doctor.
- Do not stop taking this drug abruptly; it must be discontinued gradually.
- Do not take any nonprescription preparations for cough, cold, allergy, weight loss, or sinus problems without consulting your doctor.

Medical Tests:

- Xanax may interfere with the results of some medical tests.

- Your doctor may want to conduct blood cell counts and liver function tests to monitor your progress on this drug.
- Any drug may affect the results and accuracy of a medical test. If a doctor recommends a medical or laboratory test for any condition, inform the doctor that you are taking this drug.

ZANTAC

Ingredient(s): ranitidine

Equivalent Product(s): none

Used for: treatment of active duodenal ulcer as well as conditions caused by excessive stomach acid secretion

Dosage Form and Strength: tablets—150 mg

Storage: Store in a tightly closed container at room temperature away from light.

Before Using This Drug, Tell Your Doctor: if you have a history of kidney or liver disease. Tell your doctor about any drugs, prescription or nonprescription, you are taking and about any allergies you have or any family history of allergies.

This Drug Should Not Be Used If: you are allergic to its ingredient. Otherwise, there are no known contraindications.

How to Use: Take this drug with or without food.

Time Required for Drug to Take Effect: two to three hours

Missing a Dose: Take the missed dose as soon as you remember, unless it is almost time for the next dose. In that case, do not take the missed dose, but return to your regular dosing schedule. Do not double the next dose.

Symptoms of Overdose: none known in humans. In animal studies, animals receiving large doses displayed muscle tremors, vomiting, and rapid breathing.

Side Effects:

Minor and expected:
- headache, dizziness, constipation, nausea

Serious adverse reactions (CALL YOUR DOCTOR):
- abdominal pain, rash, unusual bleeding or bruising

Effects of Long-Term Use: Studies have not been done to assess long-term use.

Habit-Forming Possibility: none

Precautions and Suggestions:

Foods and beverages:
- Ask your doctor about the most effective diet and whether you can drink alcoholic beverages.

Other medicines, prescription and nonprescription:
- To date, no drug interactions with Zantac have been reported.

Other:
- If this drug makes you dizzy, avoid activities that require alertness, such as driving a car or operating potentially dangerous machinery.
- Take Zantac consistently for as long as your doctor prescribes; do not stop taking the drug without your doctor's approval.

Medical Tests:

- Zantac may interfere with the results of a test for urine protein.
- Any drug may affect the results and accuracy of a medical test. If a doctor recommends a medical or laboratory test for any condition, inform the doctor that you are taking this drug.

ZYLOPRIM

Ingredient(s): allopurinol

Equivalent Product(s): allopurinol (generic), Lopurin

Used for: treatment of gout and prevention of excessive uric acid formation as the result of certain conditions

Dosage Form and Strength: tablets—100 mg, 300 mg

Storage: Store in a tightly closed container at room temperature.

Before Using This Drug, Tell Your Doctor: if you have blood disorders, liver or kidney disease, or if you have or any member of your family has idiopathic hemochromatosis. Tell your doctor about any drugs, prescription or nonprescription, you are taking and about any allergies you have or any family history of allergies.

This Drug Should Not Be Used If: you are allergic to its ingredient or if you have or any member of your family has idiopathic hemochromatosis.

How to Use: This drug can be taken with food to prevent stomach upset. Take each dose with a full glass of water. In addition, drink 10 to 12 full eight-ounce glasses of water a day.

Time Required for Drug to Take Effect: Body levels of uric acid may start to decrease in 48 to 72 hours, reaching a normal range in one to three weeks. However, consistent use for several months may be necessary to prevent gout attacks.

Missing a Dose: Take the missed dose as soon as you remember, unless it is almost time for the next dose. In that case, do not take the missed dose, but return to the regular dosing schedule. Do not double the next dose.

Symptoms of Overdose: No significant overdose incidents have been reported.

Side Effects:

Minor and expected:
- drowsiness, nausea, increase in acute attacks of gout at beginning of treatment (ask doctor about using another drug until this stabilizes)

Serious adverse reactions (CALL YOUR DOCTOR):
- skin rash, itching, hair loss, unusual bleeding or bruising, fever, chills, vomiting, diarrhea, abdominal pain, yellowish discoloration of skin and whites of eyes, blurred vision, joint pain, painful or difficult urination

Effects of Long-Term Use: none known

Habit-Forming Possibility: none

Precautions and Suggestions:

Foods and beverages:
- Your doctor may recommend a special diet to control your gout condition.
- Do not take large doses of vitamin C, which may increase the possibility of kidney stone formation.
- Ask your doctor if you can drink alcoholic beverages.

Other medicines, prescription and nonprescription:
- Zyloprim may increase the effects of anticoagulants and theophylline.
- Zyloprim may also interact with diuretics, mercaptopurine, azathioprine, other gout drugs (uricosurics), and some oral antidiabetes drugs.
- Zyloprim may cause excessive buildup of iron in the body if taken with iron supplements or preparations.

Other:

- Do not stop taking this drug even if your symptoms disappear.
- Do not change the dosage recommended by your doctor.
- If this drug makes you drowsy, do not engage in activities that require alertness, such as driving a car or operating potentially dangerous machinery.

Medical Tests:

- Your doctor may want to perform laboratory tests, particularly blood counts and liver and kidney function tests, to monitor your progress on this drug.
- Any drug may affect the results and accuracy of a medical test. If a doctor recommends a medical or laboratory test for any condition, inform the doctor that you are taking this drug.

11
NONPRESCRIPTION DRUGS

AFRIN

Ingredient(s): oxymetazoline hydrochloride

Equivalent Product(s): Bayfrin, Dristan Long Lasting, Duramist Plus, Duration, 4-Way Long Acting Nasal, Neo-Synephrine 12 Hour, Nostrilla, NTZ Long Acting Nasal Drops, oxymetazoline (generic), Sinex Long-Lasting

Used for: temporary relief of stuffy nose

Dosage Form and Strength: solution—0.025%, 0.05%

Storage: Store at room temperature.

This Drug Should Not Be Used If: you are allergic to its ingredient or to other decongestants or have a history of severe high blood pressure or severe coronary artery disease. You should not use this product if you are taking monoamine oxidase inhibitors. This drug should be used with caution by persons with heart disease, angina, high blood pressure, coronary artery disease, overactive thyroid gland, glaucoma, enlarged prostate gland, ulcers, or diabetes.

How to Use: Drop two or three drops or spray into each nostril in the morning and in the evening. Do not use for more than three days in a row; using this product longer may worsen the stuffiness.

Missing a Dose: Take the missed dose and then wait for about 12 hours to take the next dose. Maintain the new schedule.

Side Effects:

Minor and expected:
- stinging, burning, sneezing, dry nose, headache, rapid heartbeat

Serious adverse reactions (CALL YOUR DOCTOR):
- chronic swelling of membranes of the nose after prolonged or excessive use; also, sweating, drowsiness, deep sleep or sleeplessness, tremor, nervousness, dizziness, heartbeat irregularities, convulsions, fear, restlessness, eye tearing, sensitivity to light, weakness, difficult urination, nausea

Effects of Long-Term Use: See "Serious adverse reactions" above; also, possible mental changes and a tolerance to the drug, especially in the elderly

Habit-Forming Possibility: none

Precautions and Suggestions:

- People over the age of 60 are more likely to experience adverse reactions. Overdose in this age group may cause convulsions and hallucinations and may be very serious.
- Do not use this solution in sprayers or containers with parts made of aluminum, which reacts with the drug.
- Discoloration of the product means that it has decomposed. Discard it.
- Don't allow more than one person to use the same container.
- Rinse dropper or spray tip in hot water after each use.
- This product may interact with monoamine oxidase inhibitors, beta blockers, and some high blood pressure medications.

BENYLIN

Ingredient(s): diphenhydramine hydrochloride

Equivalent Product(s): Benadryl

Used for: control of cough, allergy-related itching and swelling of skin, motion sickness, parkinsonism

Dosage Form and Strength: syrup—12.5 mg per 5 ml

Storage: Store at room temperature.

This Drug Should Not Be Used If: you are allergic to its ingredient, have a history of heart disease or ulcers, or have asthma or another lower respiratory tract condition, glaucoma, enlarged prostate gland, or urinary obstruction. This drug should not be used by people taking monoamine oxidase inhibitors. This drug should be used with caution by those with a history of asthma, urine retention, glaucoma, overactive thyroid gland, or high blood pressure.

How to Use: Take two to four medical teaspoons (25 to 50 mg) four times a day, not to exceed 200 mg in 24 hours. Take the dose with water, food, or milk to reduce stomach upset. As a sleep aid, take four medical teaspoons (50 mg) at bedtime.

Missing a Dose: Take the missed dose as soon as possible. If it is almost time for the next dose, however, omit the missed dose and return to the regular schedule.

Side Effects:

Minor and expected:
- dry mouth, nose, or throat; dizziness; drowsiness; sensitivity to sunlight; nasal congestion; thickening of lung secretions; wheezing; headache; frequent urination; upset stomach; vomiting; diarrhea; constipation

Serious adverse reactions (CALL YOUR DOCTOR):
- excited state, rash, chills, painful or difficult urination, blurred vision, pounding heartbeat, confusion, clumsiness, unexplained sore throat, severe headache, fever, tightness in chest, tingling and weakness in the hands, convulsions, tremor, nervousness, blurred vision, ringing in the ears, insomnia, elation, delusions, impotence

Effects of Long-Term Use: This drug should not be used for a long period of time. Long-term use can lead to anemia, a deficiency of red blood cells.

Habit-Forming Possibility: none

Precautions and Suggestions:

- A persistent cough may be a sign of a serious illness. If your cough lasts longer than one week, stop taking this medication and call your doctor.
- Take this and any cough preparation only if it is really needed—as when, for example, you cannot sleep because of constant coughing. A cough is a defense mechanism and should be allowed to occur if it does not cause undue discomfort.
- If you become drowsy, do not engage in activities that require alertness.
- Do not take Benylin at the same time you are taking a sedative or tranquilizer.
- Benylin may interact with monoamine oxidase inhibitors, sedatives, tranquilizers, sleeping aids, antidepressants, and epinephrine.
- Avoid alcohol.

DIMETANE

Ingredient(s): phenylephrine hydrochloride, brompheniramine maleate

Equivalent Product(s): none

Used for: relief of symptoms accompanying upper respiratory conditions, such as runny or stuffy nose, congestion, watering eyes

Dosage Form and Strength: elixir—5 mg phenylephrine hydrochloride, 2 mg brompheniramine maleate, 2.3% alcohol; tablets—10 mg phenylephrine, 4 mg brompheniramine maleate

Storage: Store at room temperature.

This Drug Should Not Be Used If: you are allergic to its ingredients or have a history of high blood pressure. This drug should be used with caution by persons with asthma, heart disease, thyroid disease, glaucoma, enlarged prostate gland, urinary obstruction, or diabetes. This drug should be used with caution by persons taking monoamine oxidase inhibitors and/or high blood pressure medication.

How to Use:
- *Elixir*: Take two teaspoons every four hours, not to exceed 12 teaspoons in 24 hours.
- *Tablets*: Take one tablet every four hours, not to exceed six tablets in 24 hours.

Missing a Dose: Take the missed dose when you remember and then wait four hours to take the next dose. Maintain this new schedule.

Side Effects:

Minor and expected:
- drowsiness

Serious adverse reactions (CALL YOUR DOCTOR):
- nervousness, dizziness, sleeplessness, excitability

Effects of Long-Term Use: Using this drug for more than three to five days may cause the symptoms it is intended to relieve to worsen instead.

Habit-Forming Possibility: none

Precautions and Suggestions:
- If this drug causes you to become drowsy, do not engage in any activities that require alertness.
- Avoid alcohol.
- This drug may interact with monoamine oxidase inhibitors or high blood pressure medication.

DRAMAMINE

Ingredient(s): dimenhydrinate

Equivalent Product(s): Calm X, dimenhydrinate (generic), Dimentabs, Dramaban, Marmine, Motion-Aid

Used for: prevention and treatment of nausea and vomiting of motion sickness

Dosage Form and Strength: tablets—50 mg; liquid—12.5 mg per 4 ml

Storage: Store at room temperature.

This Drug Should Not Be Used If: you are allergic to its ingredient or have a history of asthma, ulcers, or heart disease.

How to Use: Take one to two tablets every four to six hours, not to exceed eight tablets in 24 hours. Two tablets may make you drowsy; do not drive in this condition. Take first dose one half hour before starting activity.

Missing a Dose: Take the missed dose when you remember unless it is almost time for the next dose. In that case, skip the missed dose and return to regular dosing schedule. Do not exceed the daily limits.

Side Effects:

Minor and expected:
- drowsiness

Serious adverse reactions (CALL YOUR DOCTOR):
- nervousness, confusion, headache, sleeplessness, heaviness and weakness of hands, nausea, vomiting, diarrhea, constipation, upset stomach, blurred vision, rash, heartbeat iregularities, stuffy nose, wheezing, tightness in chest, dry mouth and throat

Effects of Long-Term Use: not applicable

Habit-Forming Possibility: none

Precautions and Suggestions:
- This drug can react with certain antibiotics. Talk to your doctor if you are taking an antibiotic and want to take this medication.
- If you become drowsy, do not engage in any activities that require alertness, such as driving a car or operating potentially dangerous machinery.

GELUSIL

Ingredient(s): aluminum hydroxide, magnesium hydroxide, simethicone

Equivalent Product(s): Almacone II, Maalox Plus, Mylanta-II

Used for: relief of symptoms of heartburn, sour stomach, acid indigestion with gas; also provides symptomatic relief of excess stomach acid associated with ulcers, hiatal hernia, and other disorders of the gastrointestinal tract

Dosage Form and Strength: tablets—200 mg aluminum hydroxide, 200 mg magnesium hydroxide, 25 mg simethicone; 300 mg aluminum hydroxide, 200 mg magnesium hydroxide, 25 mg simethicone (called Gelusil-M); 400 mg aluminum hydroxide, 400 mg magnesium hydroxide, 30 mg simethicone (called Gelusil-II); liquid—200 mg aluminum hydroxide, 200 mg magnesium hydroxide, 25 mg simethicone; 300 mg aluminum hydroxide, 200 mg magnesium hydroxide, 25 mg simethicone (called Gelusil-M); 400 mg aluminum hydroxide, 400 mg magnesium hydroxide, 30 mg simethicone

Storage: Store at room temperature in a tightly closed container.

This Drug Should Not Be Used If: you are allergic to its ingredient, you have kidney disease, or you are taking a form of the antibiotic tetracycline.

How to Use: Take two teaspoons or tablets one hour after meals and at bedtime or as your doctor directs. Do not take more than 12 tablets or teaspoons in one 24-hour period. If you are taking Gelusil-M, do not take more than 10 tablets or teaspoons in a 24-hour period. If you are using Gelusil-II, do not use more than eight tablets or teaspoons in one 24-hour period. The tablets should be chewed and followed by a glass of water or milk.

Missing a Dose: Take the dose as soon as you remember, unless it is almost time for the next dose. In that case, skip the missed dose and return to the regular dosing schedule.

Side Effects: none known

Effects of Long-Term Use: increased body levels of magnesium and aluminum

Habit-Forming Possibility: none

Precautions and Suggestions:

- This product can prevent absorption of the antibiotic tetracycline.

- This product may also prevent the absorption of many other oral drugs, including oral anticholinergics, phenothiazine tranquilizers, digoxin, isoniazid, phenytoin, corticosteroids, quinidine, anticoagulants, and iron supplements or products.
- This product also may interact with aspirin or other salicylates and amphetamines. If you are taking any other drugs, ask your doctor if and when you can use antacids.
- This product contains small amounts of sodium; if you need to restrict sodium because of another disorder, ask your doctor if you can use Gelusil.

HYDROCORTISONE (GENERIC)

Ingredient(s): hydrocortisone acetate

Equivalent Product(s): Caladryl, CaldeCort, Cinicort, Cortaid, Epifoam, Gynecort, Lanacort, Pharma-Cort, Resicort, Rhulicort

Used for: temporary relief of minor skin irritations, including itching; rashes; insect bites; poison ivy, sumac, and oak; and discomfort caused by soaps, detergents, cosmetics, jewelry, and clothing

Dosage Form and Strength: ointment—0.5%; cream—0.5%; lotion—0.5%; foam—aerosol, 1%

Storage: Store away from light in a tightly closed container.

This Drug Should Not Be Used If: you are allergic to its ingredient or to any steroid drugs or have a fungal infection, any other infection, tuberculosis of the skin, chicken pox, shingles, herpes simplex, poor blood circulation, liver disease, or a perforated eardrum.

How to Use: Wash your hands and then wash the affected area with water. Pat dry. Apply the medication in a thin film, and rub it in lightly. Do not apply a thick layer. Do not wrap or bandage the area. If you are using the aerosol applicator, do not breathe the vapors or puncture the can. *Do not* allow the medication to get into your eyes.

Missing a Dose: Apply the missed dose as soon as you remember. If it is almost time for the next dose, however, do not apply the missed dose, but return to the original dosing schedule. *Do not* apply twice as much medication at the next dose.

Side Effects:

Minor and expected:
- a stinging, burning sensation may occur when this drug is applied; this is harmless

Serious adverse reactions (CALL YOUR DOCTOR):
- severe burning or stinging; itching, blistering, peeling, or any signs of irritation that were not present when you started to use this drug; increased hair growth; thinning of the skin; loss of skin color; signs of infection on the skin; discoloration of the skin; abnormal lines on the skin

Effects of Long-Term Use: weight gain, thinning of skin, easy bruising, loss of bone strength

Habit-Forming Possibility: There probably is none, but long-term use of a steroid drug may lead to functional dependence in which the body depends on the drug to perform a body function.

Precautions and Suggestions:
- This is a steroid drug and should be used carefully.
- Although this is a low-strength form, in order to be a nonprescription drug, you can still absorb a great deal of the medication through the skin. If the affected area does not seem to be improving, or in fact is becoming worse, discontinue use of the product and consult your doctor.

METAMUCIL

Ingredient(s): psyllium hydrophilic mucilloid and carbohydrate (differs from dosage form to dosage form) are the basic ingredients; each dosage form may have additional ingredients (see "Dosage form and strength")

Equivalent Product(s): none

Used for: management of chronic constipation, irritable bowel syndrome, and other forms of constipation arising from specific disorders

Dosage Form and Strength: powder—3.4 g psyllium and 3.5 g carbohydrate (dextrose), 1 mg sodium, 31 mg potassium; 3.4 g psyllium, 7.1 g carbohydrate (sucrose) and citric acid, 1 mg sodium, 31 mg potassium; effervescent powder—3.6 g psyllium, 0.9 g carbohydrate (sucrose) with citric acid, calcium carbonate, potassium bicarbonate, and sodium bicarbonate, 7 mg sodium, 60 mg calcium, 280 mg potassium; 3.6 g psyllium, 1.1 g carbohydrate (sucrose) with citric acid, potassium bicarbonate, sodium bicarbonate, 6 mg sodium, 307 mg potassium

Storage: Store in a tightly closed container at room temperature.

This Drug Should Not Be Used If: you have an intestinal obstruction, fecal impaction, or an allergy to its ingredients. If you should be restricting sodium or potassium because of other conditions or medications, ask your doctor about using Metamucil.

How to Use: Take one rounded teaspoon or one packet in an eight-ounce glass of cool water one to three times a day, depending on need. Drink another glass of water immediately afterward.

Missing a Dose: not applicable

Side Effects:

Minor and expected:
- excessive bowel activity, irritation at the anal opening

Serious adverse reactions (CALL YOUR DOCTOR):
- weakness, dizziness, fainting, muscle cramps, palpitations, sweating, abdominal pain, nausea, vomiting, gastrointestinal obstruction, redness or swelling of face

Effects of Long-Term Use: disruption of fluid-mineral balance in the body; possible laxative dependence

Habit-Forming Possibility: possible dependence, although this bulk form laxative is considered to be the most natural and thus to cause the least side effects

Precautions and Suggestions:

- If you have kidney disease, heart disease, edema, high blood pressure, or a gastrointestinal disorder, ask your doctor if you can use Metamucil.
- If you develop rectal bleeding or if you do not respond to this preparation, consult your doctor.
- If you are taking salicylates, nitrofurantoin, or digitalis or other heart drugs, you should not use Metamucil without approval from your doctor.

NEOSPORIN

Ingredient(s): polymyxin B, bacitracin zinc, neomycin sulfate

Equivalent Product(s): none

Used for: first aid to treat or prevent surface bacterial infections of minor cuts, scrapes, or abrasions of the skin

Dosage Form and Strength: ointment—5,000 units polymyxin, 400 units bacitracin, 5 mg neomycin per gram

Storage: Cap the tube tightly and store at room temperature.

This Drug Should Not Be Used If: you have an allergy to any of its ingredients or to any other topical antibiotic.

How to Use: Gently wash the affected area and apply the ointment in a thin layer two to five times a day at relatively evenly spaced intervals. Cover the area with sterile gauze if desired. Remove any crusting of the sore area before applying the ointment.

Missing a Dose: Apply the missed dose as soon as you remember and repeat applications after the usual intervals.

Side Effects:

Minor and expected:
- minor irritation of skin

Serious adverse reactions (CALL YOUR DOCTOR):
- swelling, scaling, itching, redness of the skin; persisting or increasing pain at the site; failure of the infection or wound to heal. Neomycin absorbed through large areas of damaged skin may lead to kidney problems or hearing difficulties.

Effects of Long-Term Use: none known

Habit-Forming Possibility: none

Precautions and Suggestions:

- This drug is not intended to be used for deep puncture wounds, serious burns, deep infections of the skin, or severe cases of impetigo. If any of these conditions applies to you, see your doctor for more appropriate treatment and/or medicine.
- Neosporin ointment must not be used in the eyes.
- If you have any doubts about how you are reacting to this medication, call your doctor.

NEO-SYNEPHRINE

Ingredient(s): phenylephrine

Equivalent Product(s): Alconefrin, Allerest, Coricidin Nasal Mist, doktors Nose Drops, Duration Mild, Newphrine, Nostril, Pyracort-D, Rhinall, Sinarest Nasal, Sinex, Sinophen Intranasal, Super Anahist

Used for: temporary relief of stuffy nose

Dosage Form and Strength: solution—0.125%, 0.25%, 0.5%, 1%

Storage: Store at room temperature.

This Drug Should Not Be Used If: you are allergic to its ingredient or have a history of severe high blood pressure or severe coronary artery disease. You should not use this product if you are taking monoamine oxidase inhibitors. This drug should be used with caution by persons with heart disease, angina, high blood pressure, coronary artery disease, overactive thyroid gland, glaucoma, enlarged prostate gland, ulcers, or diabetes.

How to Use: Place the recommended number of drops in each nostril every three to four hours. Start with the 0.25% solution; the 0.5% and 1% solutions may be needed for resistant cases. Do not use for more than three days in a row; using this product longer may worsen stuffiness.

Missing a Dose: Take the missed dose and then wait three or four hours to take the next dose. Maintain the new schedule.

Side Effects:

Minor and expected:
- stinging, burning, sneezing, dry nose, headache

Serious adverse reactions (CALL YOUR DOCTOR):
- chronic swelling of the membranes of the nose after prolonged or excessive use; sweating, drowsiness, heartbeat irregularities, weakness, tremor, convulsions, fear, restlessness, eye tearing, sensitivity to light, difficulty with urination, nausea

Effects of Long-Term Use: see "Serious adverse reactions" above; also, possible mental changes and a tolerance to the drug, especially in elderly people

Habit-Forming Possibility: none

Precautions and Suggestions:

- People over the age of 60 are more likely to experience adverse effects. Overdose in this age group may cause convulsions and hallucinations and may be very serious.
- Discoloration of this product means it has decomposed. Discard it.
- Don't allow more than one person to use the same container of Neo-Synephrine.
- Rinse the dropper or spray tip in hot water after each use.
- This product may interact with monoamine oxidase inhibitors, beta blockers, and some high blood pressure medications.

NEO-SYNEPHRINE II

Ingredient(s): xylometazoline hydrochloride

Equivalent Product(s): Chlorohist-LA, Corimist, Otrivin, Sinutab Long-Lasting, xylometazoline hydrochloride (generic)

Used for: temporary relief of stuffy nose

Dosage Form and Strength: solution—0.5%, 0.1%

Storage: Store at room temperature.

This Drug Should Not Be Used If: you are allergic to its ingredient or have a history of severe high blood pressure or severe coronary artery disease. You should not use this product if you are taking monoamine oxidase inhibitors. This drug should be used with caution by persons with heart disease, angina, high blood pressure, coronary artery disease, overactive thyroid gland, glaucoma, enlarged prostate gland, ulcers, or diabetes.

How to Use: Place two or three drops or sprays in each nostril every eight to ten hours. Do not use for more than three days in a row; using this product longer may worsen the stuffiness.

Missing a Dose: Take the missed dose and then wait eight to ten hours to take the next dose. Maintain the new schedule.

Side Effects:

Minor and expected:
- stinging, burning, sneezing, dry nose, headache, rapid heartbeat

Serious adverse reactions (CALL YOUR DOCTOR):
- chronic swelling of membranes of the nose after prolonged or excessive use, sweating, drowsiness, deep sleep or sleeplessness, nervousness, dizziness, heartbeat irregularities, weakness, tremor, convulsions, fear, restlessness, eye tearing, sensitivity to light, difficulty with urination.

Effects of Long-Term Use: see "Serious adverse reactions" above; also, possible mental changes and a tolerance to the drug, especially in the elderly

Habit-Forming Possibility: none

Precautions and Suggestions:
- People over the age of 60 are more likely to experience adverse effects. Overdose in this age group may cause convulsions and hallucinations and may be very serious.
- Do not use this solution in sprayers or containers with any parts made of aluminum, which reacts with the drug.
- Discoloration of the product means it has decomposed and should be discarded.
- Don't allow more than one person to use the same container of medication.
- Rinse the dropper or spray tip in hot water after each use.
- This product may interact with monoamine oxidase inhibitors, beta blockers, some high blood pressure medications, and diabetes drugs.

NUPRIN

Ingredient(s): ibuprofen

Equivalent Product(s): Advil (Ibuprofen is also available in higher strengths as the prescription drugs Motrin and Rufen.)

Used for: relief of mild pain associated with arthritis, headache, toothache, muscle aches, backache, menstruation, and the common cold, as well as for the reduction of fever

Dosage Form and Strength: tablets—200 mg

Storage: Store at room temperature and avoid unusually high heat (over 104 degrees Fahrenheit).

This Drug Should Not Be Used If: you are allergic or sensitive to aspirin or have ever had an allergic reaction to ibuprofen. Do not use this drug if you have nasal polyps, a history of ulcers or other stomach problems; kidney, liver, or heart disease; high blood pressure; bleeding or clotting problems. If you are taking any other medicines (prescription or nonprescription), ask your doctor if it is all right to take Nuprin at the same time. Also, if you are under a doctor's care for a serious condition, check with your doctor before taking this medicine.

How to Use: Take one or two tablets on an empty stomach one-half to one hour before or two hours after eating. However, if upset stomach occurs, take the drug with food or milk. Although the drug works faster when taken on an empty stomach, in the long run it is just as effective if taken with food or milk. Take every four to six hours.

Time Required for Drug to Take Effect: Nuprin takes effect within one hour, and its benefits continue for three to five hours.

Missing a Dose: Take the missed dose as soon as you remember and then continue with the usual schedule. However, if it is nearly time for the next dose, skip the missed dose and return to the usual schedule. Do not double the dose.

Side Effects:

Minor and expected:
- indigestion, nausea, cramping, excessive gas, bloating, diarrhea, constipation, headache, nervousness, loss of appetite

Serious adverse reactions (CALL YOUR DOCTOR):
- blurred, diminished, and/or changed vision; skin rash; hives; itching; fluid retention resulting in weight gain; bloody or black, tarry stools; ringing in the ears; yellowish skin or eyes; decreased hearing; pounding heartbeat; confusion; chills; difficult breathing; unexplained sore throat; fever

Effects of Long-Term Use: possible harmful effect on kidney or liver function

Habit-Forming Possibility: none known

Precautions and Suggestions:

- Avoid alcohol since the combination of ibuprofen and alcohol can increase the possibility of stomach irritation and bleeding.

- Do not take aspirin at the same time you are taking Nuprin.
- This drug may interact with phenobarbital, phenytoin (Dilantin), sulfa drugs, pain medications, and some high blood pressure medicines.
- Nuprin's ability to reduce both inflammation and fever can conceal signs of infection. If you develop any symptoms that may indicate a new or unrelated condition or illness, call your doctor.

ROBITUSSIN

Ingredient(s): guaifenesin

Equivalent Product(s): Anti-Tuss, Baytussin, Colrex, Cremacoat 2 Liquid, GG-CEN, Glyate, Glycotuss, guaifenesin (generic), Guiamid, Guiatuss, Halotussin, Malotuss, Nortussin, Peedee Dose Expectorant, Robafen, S-T Expectorant SF & DF

Used for: relief of dry, nonproductive cough

Dosage Form and Strength: syrup—100 mg per 5 ml

Storage: Store this drug at room temperature.

This Drug Should Not Be Used If: you are allergic to its ingredient. This product should not be used for a chronic cough (such as that caused by asthma, emphysema, or smoking) or for a cough that produces a great amount of secretions. You should not take this medication if you have a high fever, persistent headache, rash, nausea, or vomiting. If those symptoms are present, call your doctor.

How to Use: Take 1 to 4 teaspoons every 4 hours, not to exceed 24 teaspoons in 24 hours. It is best to try to give the smallest dosage at first to see if you can get by with less medication.

Missing a Dose: Give the missed dose and then wait four hours to give the next dose. Maintain the new schedule.

Side Effects:

Minor and expected:
- drowsiness

Serious adverse reactions (CALL YOUR DOCTOR):
- nausea, vomiting, upset stomach

Effects of Long-Term Use: not applicable

Habit-Forming Possibility: none

Precautions and Suggestions:

- A persistent cough may be a sign of a serious illness. If the cough lasts longer than one week, stop taking this medication and call your doctor.
- Take this and any cough preparations only if really needed, as, for example, when you cannot sleep because of constant coughing. A cough is a defense mechanism and should be allowed to occur if it does not cause undue discomfort.

ROMILAR CF 8 HOUR COUGH FORMULA

Ingredient(s): dextromethorphan

Equivalent Product(s): Pertussin 8 Hour Cough Formula

Used for: controlling coughing

Dosage Form and Strength: syrup—15 mg per 5 ml

Storage: Store at room temperature.

This Drug Should Not Be Used If: you are allergic to its ingredient. This product should not be used for a chronic cough (such as that caused by asthma, emphysema, or smoking) or for a cough that produces a great amount of secretions. You should not take this medication if you have a high fever, persistent headache, rash, nausea, or vomiting. Call your doctor if these conditions exist. This drug should not be used by anyone taking monoamine oxidase inhibitors.

How to Use: Take two teaspoons every four to eight hours. Do not exceed eight teaspoons in 24 hours.

Missing a Dose: Take the missed dose and then wait four to eight hours to take the next dose. Increasing the dose or taking doses close together increases the action of the drug, which is not advisable in older persons.

Side Effects:

Minor and expected:
- drowsiness, nausea, vomiting

Serious adverse reactions (CALL YOUR DOCTOR):
- none known

Effects of Long-Term Use: not applicable

Habit-Forming Possibility: none

Precautions and Suggestions:

- A persistent cough may be a sign of a serious illness. If the cough lasts longer than one week, stop taking this medication and call your doctor.
- Take this and any cough preparations only if really needed, as, for example, when you cannot sleep because of constant coughing. A cough is a defense mechanism and should be allowed to occur if it does not cause undue discomfort.

SUDAFED

Ingredient(s): pseudoephedrine hydrochloride

Equivalent Product(s): Cenafed, Kodet SE, Neofed, Neo-Synephrinol Day Relief, Novafed, Peedee Dose Decongestant, pseudoephedrine (generic), Sudrin

Used for: temporary relief of stuffy nose

Dosage Form and Strength: tablets—30 mg, 60 mg; liquid—30 mg per 5 ml; capsules, timed-release—120 mg

Storage: Store at room temperature in a dry, dark place.

This Drug Should Not Be Used If: you are allergic to its ingredient or have a history of severe high blood pressure or severe coronary artery disease. You should not use this product if you are taking monoamine oxidase inhibitors. This drug should be used with caution by persons with heart disease, angina, high blood pressure, coronary artery disease, overactive thyroid gland, glaucoma, enlarged prostate gland, ulcers, or diabetes.

How to Use: Take 60 mg every six hours, not to exceed 240 mg in 24 hours. If you are using the timed-release capsule, take one capsule every 12 hours. If symptoms do not improve within seven days or if you develop a high fever, discontinue using the medication and call your doctor.

Missing a Dose: Take the missed dose and then wait 6 hours (or 12 hours if taking timed-release capsule) to take the next dose. Maintain the new schedule.

Side Effects:

Minor and expected:
- stinging or burning in nose, sneezing, dry nose, headache, drowsiness, headache, rapid heartbeat

Serious adverse reactions (CALL YOUR DOCTOR):
- sweating, deep sleep or sleeplessness, nervousness, dizziness, heartbeat irregularities, weakness, convulsions, fear, restlessness, tremor, eye tearing, sensitivity to light, difficulty with urination, nausea

Effects of Long-Term Use: not applicable since you should not use it for more than seven days

Habit-Forming Possibility: none

Precautions and Suggestions:

- Do not exceed recommended dosages.
- Oral nasal decongestants are usually not as effective as nose drops, but they are active longer and have not been found to cause increased stuffiness.
- People over the age of 60 are more likely to experience adverse effects. Overdose in this age group may be very serious.
- This product may interact with monoamine oxidase inhibitors or some high blood pressure medications.

INDEX